Intr
Care
MRC
Beyond

Published titles in the MRCOG and Beyond series

Antenatal Disorders for the MRCOG and Beyond *by Andrew Thomson and Ian Greer*

Fetal Medicine for the MRCOG and Beyond *by Alan Cameron, Lena Macara, Janet Brennand and Peter Milton*

Gynaecological and Obstetric Pathology for the MRCOG *by Harold Fox and C. Hilary Buckley, with a chapter on Cervical Cytology by Dulcie V. Coleman*

Management of Infertility for the MRCOG and Beyond *by Allan A. Templeton et al.*

Menopause for the MRCOG and Beyond *by Margaret Rees*

Menstrual Problems for the MRCOG *by Mary Ann Lumsden, Jane Norman and Hilary Critchley*

Neonatology for the MRCOG *by Peter Dear and Simon Newell*

The MRCOG: A Guide to the Examination *by Ian Johnson et al.*

Forthcoming titles in the series

Early Pregnancy Issues

Gynaecological Oncology

Gynaecological Urology

Molecular Medicine

Reproductive Endocrinology

Intrapartum Care

Thomas F. Baskett MB, FRCS(C), FRCS(Ed), FRCOG
Professor, Department of Obstetrics and Gynaecology,
Dalhousie University, Halifax, Nova Scotia, Canada

Sabaratnam Arulkumaran MB, PhD, FRCS (Ed), FRCOG
Professor and Head, Department of Obstetrics and
Gynaecology, St. George's Hospital Medical School,
London, UK

With a chapter on Neonatal Resuscitation
by John McIntyre MD MRCP MD, MRCP
Senior Lecturer and Consultant, Derby City General Hospital, Derby, UK

And a chapter on Perinatal Loss
by Carolyn Basak RN, RM, ADM, BSc, PGCEA
Senior Lecturer in Midwifery and Women's Health, Faculty of Health
and Social Care Sciences, Kingston University and St George's Medical
School, London, UK

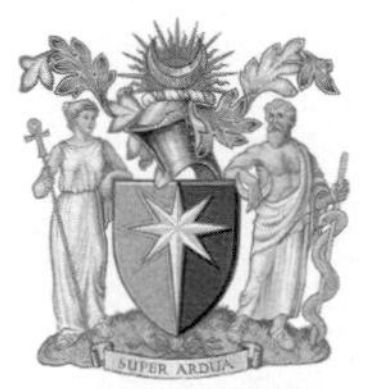

RCOG Press

First published 2002

ISBN 1-900364-73-5

Published by the **RCOG Press** at
The Royal College of Obstetricians and Gynaecologists
27 Sussex Place, Regent's Park
London NW1 4RG

Registered charity no. 213280

Line drawings by Oxford Designers and Illustrators © RCOG
Cover illustration: A caesarean section operation in progress

RCOG Editor: Jane Moody
Index: Liza Furnival
Printed by Cambrian Printers, Llanbadarn Road, Aberystwyth, Ceredigion SY23 3TN.

Contents

Preface

The labour ward is still considered by many to be the 'front line' of our profession. Indeed, it is while managing the labour ward that we will be required in a very short space of time to make important decisions that may have a vast impact on the health or even the life of a mother or her unborn child. However, this stressful and potentially litigious environment can often be one of the most enjoyable aspects of the profession. With the shortening of the number of hours per week that trainees may work, and the number of years to achieve consultant status, clinicians can no longer assume that they will be familiar with whatever they face when they take charge of the labour ward. It is vitally important that all those who are involved in the intrapartum care of women are familiar almost to the point of tedium with the procedures necessary to deal with obstetric emergencies and complications.

This book is intended to give an outline of the problems that may be encountered and their management. As such, it is a comprehensive *aide-mémoire* and forms the basis of knowledge that would be expected of any membership candidate. However, it does not replace the knowledge gained from practical experience of facing the problems first-hand.

Karl S. Oláh
Publications Editorial Committee 1997–1999
June 2002

Abbreviations

AFE	amniotic fluid embolism
bpm	beats per minute
COX	cyclo-oxygenase
CTG	cardiotocography
DIC	disseminated intravascular coagulation
ECG	electrocardiogram
EFM	electronic fetal heart rate monitoring
FBS	fetal blood sampling
IUGR	intrauterine growth restriction
MRI	magnetic resonance imaging
OA	occipitoanterior
OP	occipitoposterior
OT	occipitotransverse
PPH	postpartum haemorrhage
PROM	prelabour rupture of the membranes
Rh	rhesus
USP	United States Pharmacopeia

Introduction

Pregnancy and childbirth carry risks for the mother and to her baby. Worldwide, some 600 000 maternal deaths are recorded each year, of which 99% occur in developing countries. Many developed countries such as the United Kingdom record low maternal mortality rates of about six per 100 000 and perinatal mortality rates of 6–8 per 1000. However, the Confidential Enquiries into Maternal Deaths in the United Kingdom and the Confidential Enquiries into Stillbirths and Deaths in Infancy continue to demonstrate avoidable factors in many maternal and perinatal deaths. Because maternal mortality rates are low, obstetric units are encouraged to audit the standard of maternal care by reviewing all cases of severe maternal morbidity, often called 'near-miss' mortality. Depending on definitions, there are approximately 20–30 near-miss cases per maternal death. Similarly, the perinatal risk is greatest during labour and delivery and standards of perinatal care can be assessed by reviews of perinatal mortality and morbidity, including asphyxia, trauma and infection.

Medical and nursing staff who care for women in labour have to balance these genuine but relatively rare risks during labour and delivery with the parents' individual wishes for their own care. As outlined in the *Changing Childbirth* report (Department of Health 1993), this requires a coordinated effort to provide the best intrapartum care with a blend of evidence-based medicine, good nursing and medical knowledge, available facilities and the wishes of the woman.

Towards Safer Childbirth, the report produced by a joint working party of the Royal College of Obstetricians and Gynaecologists and Royal College of Midwives (1999) reviews the problems raised by the Confidential Enquiries into Maternal Deaths and Stillbirths and Deaths in Infancy. This report, which should be read by all those who provide intrapartum care, outlines the facilities and staffing requirements, the need for continuing medical and nursing education including 'practice runs' for intrapartum emergencies, critical incident analysis, and easily accessible current evidence-based information.

In this book we have not approached each chapter as a comprehensive review article but aimed to provide a balanced but pragmatic guide to clinical intrapartum care.

References

Department of Health. (1993) *Changing Childbirth: Report of the Expert Maternity Group* (Chairman: Baroness Cumberlege). London: HMSO.

Royal College of Obstetricians and Gynaecologists, Royal College of Midwives. (1999) *Towards Safer Childbirth: Minimum Standards for the Organisation of Labour Wards. Report of a Joint Working Party*. London: RCOG Press.

1 First stage of labour

The first stage of labour starts with the onset of regular painful uterine contractions that lead to the progressive effacement and full dilatation of the cervix.

Diagnosis of labour

Establishing the diagnosis of labour is the most basic and essential aspect of labour-ward management. In no other branch of clinical medicine do we expect the patient to make a diagnosis upon which will be based all future management. Happily, most women who present themselves to hospital at term believing that they are in labour are correct. A presumed diagnosis of labour is based upon the onset of regular and painful contractions, which are of increasing frequency and duration. This is often associated with a bloodstained mucous 'show' and, less often, rupture of the membranes. However, for the diagnosis of labour to be clearly established, these symptoms and signs have to be associated with a significant change in effacement and dilatation of the cervix. The most important aspect is effacement of the cervix and, provided that this has occurred, together with a cervical dilatation of ≥ 2 cm, the diagnosis is confirmed. Most women believing themselves to be in labour can have this diagnosis confirmed and a smaller number can be assured that they are not in labour. There remains a group of about 10–15% in whom neither the woman nor the attendant can confirm whether or not they are in labour. In such cases, the woman should be told this and then she should be observed over the next two to six hours, with repeat assessment of the cervix, which should lead to a firm diagnosis. This period of observation should be carried out away from the active labour ward if at all possible. If an incorrect diagnosis of labour is made when the woman is only in spurious labour, a series of inappropriate interventions (amniotomy, oxytocin augmentation, operative delivery) may ensue over a long and demoralising period of time.

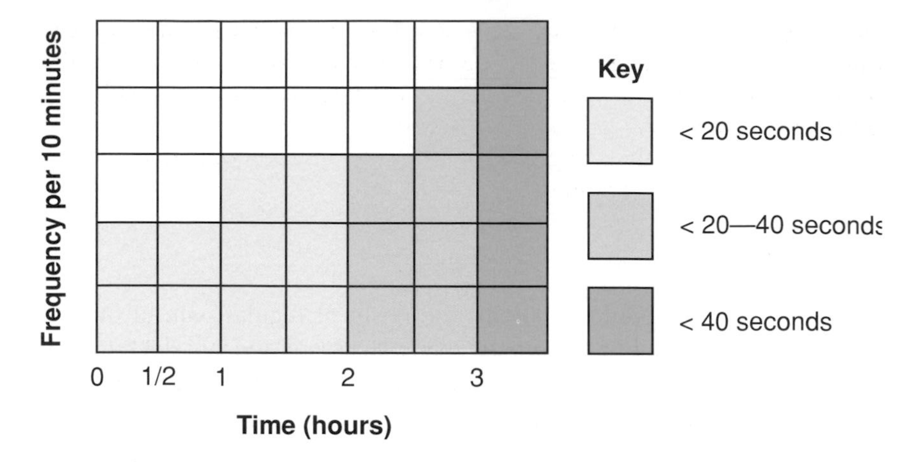

Figure 1.1 Quantification of uterine contractions by clinical palpation; frequency per ten minutes is recorded by shading the equivalent number of boxes; the type of shading indicates the duration of each contraction

Assessment of labour

There are three main components in the assessment and management of the first stage of labour. These are the progress of labour, the condition of the mother and the condition of the fetus. For the purposes of this chapter we will discuss the fetus at term in cephalic presentation.

PROGRESS OF LABOUR

Uterine contractions are recorded by their frequency, duration and strength (Figure 1.1). The state of the cervix is recorded in terms of its effacement and dilatation. In addition, other features such as anterior or mid position of the cervix in early labour, together with a soft and distensible consistency as labour progresses, are favourable signs. On the other hand, posterior position of the cervix in early labour and a thickened and oedematous consistency as labour progresses are less favourable signs.

The main function of uterine contractions in the first stage of labour is cervical effacement and dilatation. To a lesser degree there is descent of the presenting part, although the majority of descent occurs in the second stage of labour.

The position of the fetal head may be occipitoanterior, which is the most favourable, occipitotransverse or occipitoposterior. The latter two positions tend to be associated with varying degrees of deflexion, which presents a larger diameter of the fetal head to the bony pelvis. It is common to have a degree of asynclitism, such that one parietal bone presents at a higher plane than the other, with the head in the transverse position as it enters the pelvis. Anterior asynclitism is physiological but posterior asynclitism is unfavourable and may indicate disproportion.

Caput is a rather subjective assessment of the amount of oedema in the scalp soft tissues. This is rated as +, ++ or +++.

Moulding may be classified as follows:

- none Bones normally separated
- \+ Bones touching
- ++ Bones overlapping but easily separated with digital pressure
- +++ Bones overlapping and not separable with digital pressure.

The finding of + and ++ degrees of moulding is quite compatible with normal progress and vaginal delivery, whereas +++ is usually a sign of cephalopelvic disproportion.

The station of the presenting part is defined as the level of the lowest part of the fetal bony skull in relation to the ischial spines. With varying degrees of caput and moulding it can be difficult to assess the true level of the bony part in relation to the ischial spines by vaginal examination alone. Thus, a combination of vaginal assessment of the descent of the fetal head measured in centimetres above or below the ischial spines is combined with an abdominal assessment of the level of fetal head in fifths above the pelvic brim (Figure 1.2) (see Chapter 2).

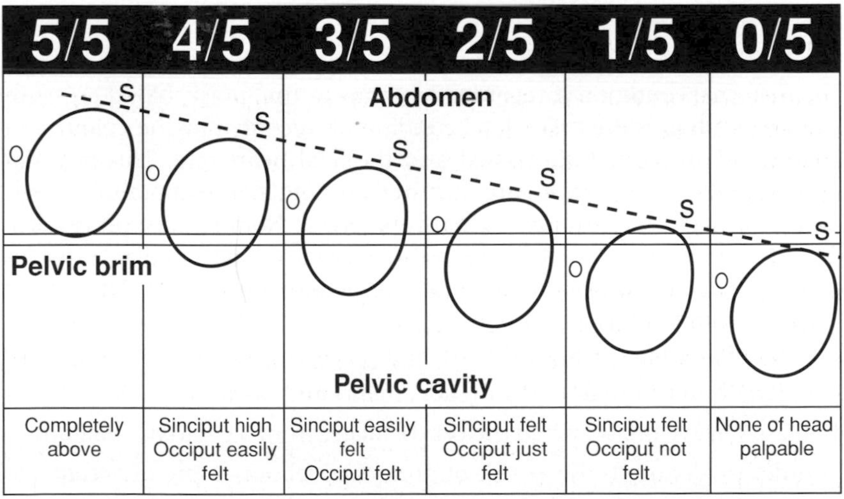

5/5	4/5	3/5	2/5	1/5	0/5
Completely above	Sinciput high Occiput easily felt	Sinciput easily felt Occiput felt	Sinciput felt Occiput just felt	Sinciput felt Occiput not felt	None of head palpable

Abdomen
Pelvic brim
Pelvic cavity

Figure 1.2 Clinical estimation of the descent of the fetal head in fifths, palpable above the pelvic brim; O = occiput; S = sinciput

Assessment of the bony pelvis during the pelvic examination, while subjective, is a worthwhile exercise and, with experience, useful clinical information can be obtained. Each attendant on the labour ward should measure their own fingers and fist, enabling them to assess some of the following aspects of the bony pelvis. The diagonal conjugate from the sacral promontory to the inner aspect of the symphysis should measure at least 12 cm. The sacrum should be nicely curved with the lower end not too prominent anteriorly. The pelvic sidewalls should be parallel rather than convergent. The prominence of the ischial spines should be noted and the sacrospinous ligaments palpated; they should accept at least two fingers (≥ 4 cm). The subpubic arch should not be unduly narrowed and the intertuberous diameter should be at least 10 cm. It is recognised that many of the above assessments are rather subjective but, with practice, individuals can gain valuable clinical experience about the bony fetopelvic relationships in labour.

CHARTING THE PROGRESS OF LABOUR

Friedman (1955) developed the basis for scientific study of the progress of labour by graphically depicting the rate of cervical dilatation against time. This cervicogram forms the basis of the modern partogram and incorporates aspects of the progress of labour, together with the condition of the mother and the fetus in a chronological manner on one page. The parameters of labour progress include:

- frequency and duration of uterine contractions
- cervical effacement and dilatation
- descent of the presenting part.

The maternal condition is recorded by temperature, pulse, blood pressure and drugs administered. The fetal condition is recorded by the colour and quantity of amniotic fluid passed and the fetal heart rate. This pictorial documentation of labour assures a systematic and logical appraisal, which facilitates early recognition of poor progress. Nomograms of cervical dilatation confirm that different ethnic groups have similar rates of cervical dilatation and uterine activity in spontaneous labour. The rate of cervical dilatation has two phases:

- a slow latent phase during which the cervix shortens from about 3 cm in length to less than 0.5 cm (effacement) and dilates to 3 cm
- a faster active phase, when the cervix dilates from 3 cm to full dilatation.

In order to identify those at risk of prolonged labour, a line of acceptable progress known as the 'alert line' is drawn on the partogram. If the rate of cervical dilatation crosses to the right of the alert line, progress is

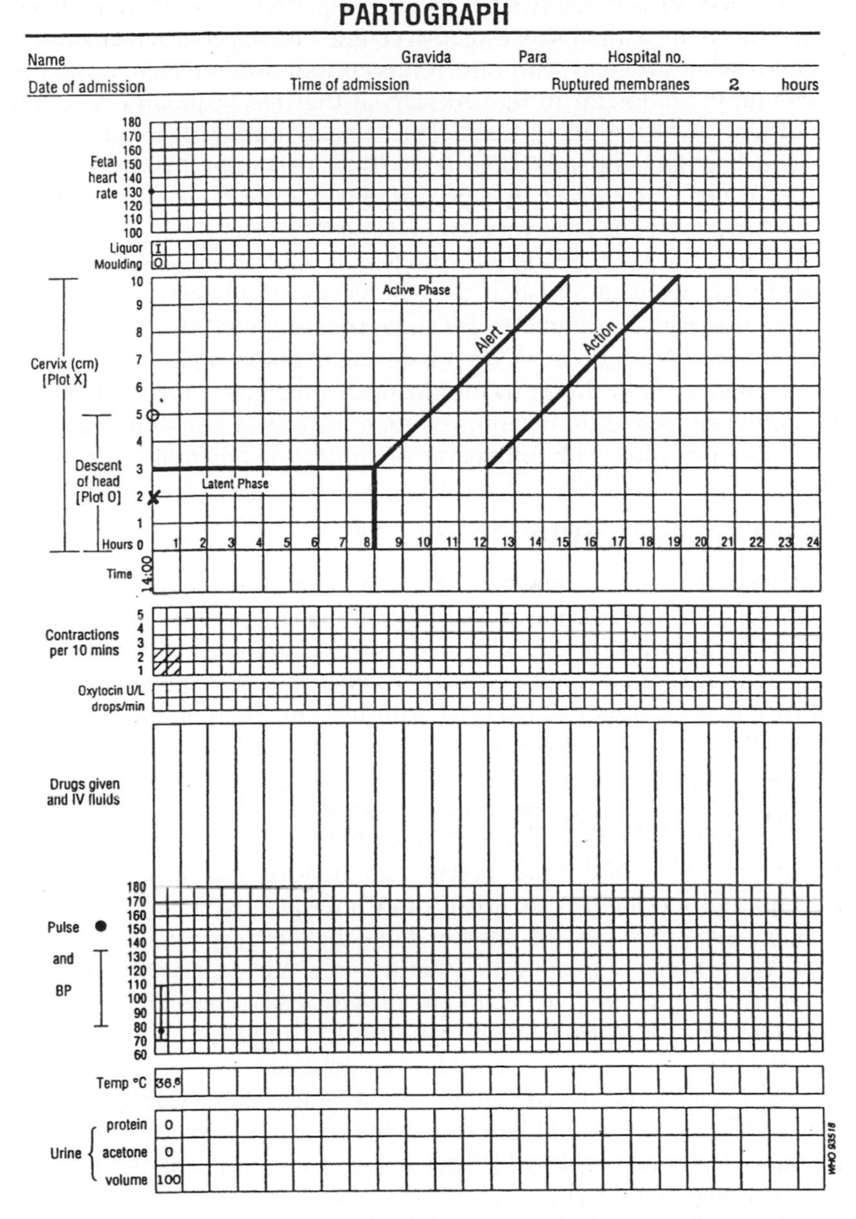

Figure 1.3 World Health Organization partograph showing alert and action lines in the latent and active phase of labour; cervical dilatation, decent of head, fetal parameters (heart rate, colour of liquor, caput and moulding), maternal parameters (pulse, blood pressure, results of urine tests and drugs used) can be entered

deemed to be unsatisfactory. The line of acceptable progress can be based on the mean, median or slowest tenth centile rate of cervical dilatation in women who progress without intervention and deliver normally. Intervention is thought to be necessary if the rate of progress cuts the 'action line', which is drawn parallel and one to four hours to the right of the alert line (Philpott and Castle 1972). Thus, depending on which of the above criteria are applied, the proportion of labours deemed to have unsatisfactory progress can vary from 5% to 50%. Each unit will develop its own principles that define non-progressive labour but the principle of partographic depiction of labour should be universally applied. This has been endorsed by the World Health Organization (1994) (Figure 1.3). The latent phase of labour may last up to eight hours in the nulliparous woman and up to six hours in multiparae. In the active phase of labour, both nulliparous and multiparous women dilate at a rate of at least one centimetre per hour, with multiparae often dilating much more rapidly.

Maternal condition

Upon admission to the labour ward, the antenatal chart is reviewed and an abbreviated history and physical examination performed. This will include temperature, pulse, blood pressure, abdominal palpation, fetal heart auscultation and urinalysis. Depending on the woman's history of uterine contractions, show and rupture of membranes, vaginal examination may be performed to confirm the diagnosis of labour or postponed until later. If the diagnosis of labour is confirmed, this should be reviewed with the woman and an optimistic approach conveyed about forthcoming events. If the woman is in early labour she may wish to have fluids and a light snack. If she is established in active labour, sips of water, ice chips and sucking hard sweets is more appropriate.

If the pregnancy is low risk and it is likely that delivery will occur within six to eight hours, an intravenous infusion is not necessary. However, should the mother require epidural analgesia, become dehydrated, or should labour be prolonged or high risk, an intravenous infusion of crystalloid or dextrose/saline should be established.

When possible, the woman should be up and walking during the first stage of labour. She should be encouraged to assume whatever position she finds most comfortable, which is usually sitting, reclining or the lateral semi-recumbent position.

No woman in labour should be left alone. While some partners are helpful during labour, they cannot replace a knowledgeable nurse/midwife. Each hospital will develop its own guidelines for the attendance of companions and family members in labour but their roles with regard to the nursing and medical staff should be clearly established.

Explanation of progress and any interventions should be carefully outlined to the woman and her partner. Although there is enormous pressure on nursing and medical staff to chart all events for audit and medico-legal purposes, a balance between this and common sense, clinical care and communication must be achieved.

Fetal condition

Generally speaking, in low-risk cases the fetus that enters labour in good condition is unlikely to suffer asphyxia during a normally progressive labour. Thus, if the fetal heart at the start of labour is normal, there is no meconium staining and the subsequent progress of labour is normal, the outlook for a delivery of a normal, well-oxygenated infant is excellent. Auscultation of the fetal heart before, during and after one contraction every 15 minutes in the first stage of labour is adequate. If the pregnancy is high risk, there is any abnormality of the fetal heart or meconium staining of the amniotic fluid, continuous electronic monitoring of the fetal heart rate is advisable. Various options should be made available: if auscultation every 15 minutes is not feasible, or at the request of the woman, a compromise is to have a 10–20 minute admission screening test with external monitoring of the fetal heart rate (Ingemarsson *et al.* 1986). If this is completely normal and the amniotic fluid is clear, then auscultation may replace the electronic fetal heart monitor if the woman wishes. The details of fetal surveillance in labour are outlined in Chapter 3.

Analgesia

Childbirth classes that include education and training for relaxation and breathing techniques help some women in labour. However, the majority, particularly primiparous women, will request additional analgesia.

Randomised trials have shown that continuous support and explanation, not always from a professional nurse, shortens labour, lessens the requirements for analgesia and reduces operative delivery (Kennell *et al.* 1991).

Systemic narcotic analgesia is most often given using pethidine (in the USA and Canada, meperidine, demerol). The dose ranges from 50–150 mg intramuscularly. It is usually given in the first stage of labour and probably has its main benefit in anxious women with a painful latent phase. It can be given in 25-mg increments intravenously every three to five minutes in order to give rapid relief in a patient in whom pain has been allowed to get out of control. Both pethidine and fentanyl have been used in an intravenous patient-controlled administration set. There is no evidence that this provides superior analgesia but it does reduce the total amount of drug given. Other than a delay in gastric emptying, which may be relevant if subsequent general anaesthesia is required, pethidine has no serious maternal adverse effects in the doses used. The main potential drawback is respiratory depression in the newborn if delivery occurs one to three hours following administration to the mother. This can be dealt with by providing assisted ventilation to the infant and administering the narcotic antagonist naloxone in a dose of 0.1 mg/kg by intramuscular injection or, if the infant requires an endotracheal tube, by this route. Pethidine may also impair the establishment of breastfeeding (Ransjö-Arvidson *et al.* 2001).

Inhalation analgesia is simple, safe and, within limits, effective. The most practical and safest is a 50% nitrous oxide and 50% oxygen mixture. This comes in a variety of devices for self-administration. There is a latent period between the woman starting inhalation and there being sufficient gas tension in the central nervous system to produce analgesia. This usually takes five to six deep breaths and it is therefore important to help the woman to start breathing the gas before she feels the pain of the uterine contraction. This can be done by timing if the contractions are regular or by the fact that a palpable uterine contraction is felt before the woman feels the pain. In general, this method of analgesia can be exhausting and dehydrating if it is used for too long. Its main benefit is for the woman, usually multiparous, in the late first stage of labour when labour is progressing rapidly and becoming very painful. It will often see the woman through the late first stage and early second stage until she can begin bearing-down efforts.

While skilfully applied narcotic and inhalation analgesia may be adequate for a number of women, particularly multiparous women, many will request epidural analgesia. Details of the administration of epidural analgesia is beyond the scope of this book but those who have worked in units with and without this service will attest to the enormous humane benefits that this technique of pain relief has brought to labour. Epidural analgesia does not interfere with progress in the first stage of labour but it can have a profound effect on the second stage and this is discussed in Chapter 2.

Management of non-progressive labour

CAUSES

It is still reasonable to consider the three Ps in the causation of non-progressive labour.

> **NON-PROGRESSIVE LABOUR: THE THREE PS**
>
> - Powers
> - Passages
> - Passenger

Often, non-progression is caused by a combination of all three. The most practical clinical approach to the 'powers' is to consider uterine action effective or ineffective depending on whether it causes appropriate dilatation of the cervix. The 'passages' are assessed clinically. In the developed world a contracted pelvis is extremely rare, but previous pelvic fractures may be relevant. Soft tissue obstruction, such as a cervical fibroid, is also rare. X-ray pelvimetry is of no help in the clinical management of non-progressive labour. The 'passenger' may be too large for the pelvis or, more frequently, the fetal head is deflexed in the occipitotransverse or occipitoposterior position. This deflexion can present as much as a 1.5-cm increased diameter to the bony pelvis. Malpresentations such as brow should also be sought. With antenatal care and ultrasound it is rare nowadays for a fetal anomaly such as hydrocephaly to be first discovered during labour.

AUGMENTATION OF LABOUR

Augmentation of the active phase of labour can be carried out by amniotomy and, if this fails, by augmentation with oxytocin. The protocol for oxytocin infusion is shown in Chapter 6. Once the partogram shows non-progressive labour, the number of women who receive augmentation depends on how quickly one feels this should be instituted. In the Dublin active management of labour approach this may be up to 55% of all nulliparous women (O'Driscoll *et al.* 1993). If a slow progress of two hours to the right of the alert line (action line) is accepted before instituting augmentation then about 20% will require augmentation (Arulkumaran *et al.* 1987). Depending upon the wishes of the woman and the staffing in various units, the action line can be one to four hours to the right when augmentation is instituted. There is no correct answer to this, but the principle of correcting inefficient uterine action with augmentation is sound. If there is delay in the early part of the active phase, 3–7 cm, this is sometimes called primary dysfunctional labour or protraction disorder. This is often a combination of relative disproportion due to deflexion of the fetal head and ineffective uterine action. Many of these cases will respond well to augmentation. Secondary arrest of labour after 7 cm may have the same genesis but is more often due to cephalopelvic disproportion (Figure 1.4). In either event, the only influence that the obstetrician can bring to bear is to improve uterine action and hope that with progressive dilatation and descent there will be flexion and rotation of the fetal head presenting a smaller diameter to the pelvis (Fitzpatrick *et al.* 2001). In the second stage of labour relative cephalopelvic disproportion due to deflexion of the occipitoposterior position may respond to flexion with forceps or vacuum rotation (see Chapter 7).

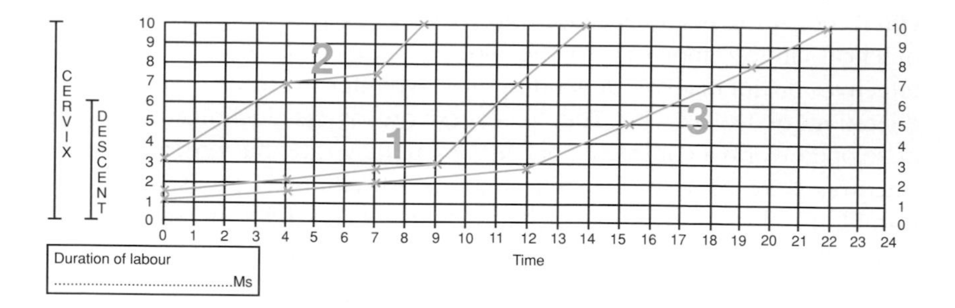

Figure 1.4 Abnormal labour patterns: (1) prolonged latent phase; (2) secondary arrest; (3) prolonged latent phase and primary dysfunctional labour

Non-progressive labour is a trying event for all concerned. Care during labour should be directed towards sustaining the morale of the woman and her partner, maintaining maternal hydration and providing adequate analgesia.

References

Arulkumaran S, Koh CH, Ingemarsson I, Ratnam SS. (1987) Augmentation of labour: Mode of delivery related to cervimetric progress. *Aust N Z J Obstet Gynaecol* 27:304–8.

Fitzpatrick M, McQuillan K, O'Herlihy C. (2001) Influence of persistent occiput posterior position on delivery outcome. *Obstet Gynecol* 98:1027–31.

Friedman EA. (1955) Primigravid labor – a graphiostatistical analysis. *Obstet Gynecol* 6:567–89.

Ingemarsson I, Arulkumaran S, Ingemarsson E. (1986) Admission test: a screening test for fetal distress in labor. *Obstet Gynecol* 68:800–6.

Kennell J, Klaus M, McGrath S. (1991) Continuous emotional support during labor in a US hospital. *JAMA* 265:2197–201.

O'Driscoll K, Meagher D, Boylan P. (1993) *Active Management of Labour*, 3rd ed. London: Mosby.

Philpott RH, Castle WM. (1972) Cervicographs in the management of labour in primigravidae I & II. *J Obstet Gynaecol Br Cwlth* 79:592–602.

Ransjö-Arvidson AB, Matthieson AS, Lilja G, Nissen E, Widström AM, Uvnäs-Moberg K. (2001) Maternal analgesia during labour disturbs newborn behaviour: effects on breastfeeding, temperature, and crying. *Birth* 28:5–12.

World Health Organization. (1994) Partograph in management of labour. *Lancet* 343:1399–404.

2 Second stage of labour

The second stage of labour lasts from full dilatation of the cervix to delivery of the infant. It is the stage when the fetus is most vulnerable, with hypoxia and trauma being the main threats. These were highlighted in the 4th Annual Report of the Confidential Inquiry into Stillbirths and Deaths in Infancy (1997), emphasising the clinical and medico-legal aspects of second stage of labour.

The second stage has two phases: the first, passive phase occurs from full dilatation of the cervix until the head descends to the pelvic floor and the second, active phase, when bearing-down efforts of the mother begin. Thus, the terms passive and active refer to maternal effort. The two phases may also be referred to as the pelvic and perineal phases. In the multiparous woman the passive phase can be very brief and last only a few minutes. However, in the nulliparous woman the head is often at the level of the ischial spines when full dilatation is reached and more time and uterine action is required to cause descent of the presenting part to the pelvic floor. In this and other aspects of care during labour, it is important to differentiate between the rate of progress of the nulliparous and multiparous woman.

Effect of epidural analgesia

The influence of epidural analgesia on the second stage of labour is relevant. In normal spontaneous labour there is an increase in the endogenous production of oxytocin in the second stage, which augments uterine action and aids descent of the presenting part. This physiological increase of oxytocin is blocked by epidural anaesthesia due to the interruption of Ferguson's reflex (Goodfellow *et al.* 1983). It is, therefore, often necessary to start or increase oxytocin augmentation during the second stage of labour when epidural analgesia is in place. Epidural anaesthesia also blunts the maternal bearing down reflex. This applies to both nulliparous and multiparous women, although with appropriate coaching the multiparous woman can usually apply adequate maternal effort in the presence of epidural anaesthesia. More sophisticated epidural techniques with selective sensory blocks are an improvement in this regard. An understanding of the effect of epidural analgesia on the second stage and the need to replace the usual physiological increase of oxytocin production can, to some extent, counteract the prolongation of the second stage and need for assisted vaginal delivery with epidural analgesia (Bates *et al.* 1985; Saunders *et al.* 1989).

Duration of labour

In most cases, the second stage of labour shows clear clinical progress with descent of the head to the pelvic floor, maternal bearing-down effort, lengthening of the perineum with contractions and gradual dilatation of the anus so that the anterior mucosa of the anal canal is seen, showing that the head is low in the pelvis.

In the normally progressive second stage of labour without epidural analgesia, most multiparous women will be delivered within 30 minutes and nulliparous women within 60 minutes. There are, however, many exceptions to this, and the length of the second stage may be influenced by parity, fetal weight, malposition of the fetal head (deflexed occipitotransverse and occipitoposterior), maternal effort, effectiveness of uterine contractions and epidural analgesia. Thus, no specific time limit is put on the duration of the second stage provided that the maternal and fetal condition are satisfactory. Such a conservative approach has not been shown to jeopardise fetal and neonatal condition, provided that the fetus is monitored appropriately (Menticoglou *et al.* 1995).

While there should be no set time limit on the duration of the second stage, guidelines to assess the progress, or lack thereof, are necessary so that appropriate intervention can be considered. There is arrest of progress in the second stage if there is no descent after 30 minutes in the multiparous woman and 60 minutes in the nulliparous. Protracted progress is less than 2-cm descent per hour in multiparous and less than 1 cm in the nulliparous woman. Most cases with inadequate progress in the second stage of labour are in the nulliparous woman. As a working guide, allow one hour after full dilatation without maternal effort and, if the head has not descended to the pelvic floor, start oxytocin augmentation. After a further hour, maternal effort should be added for the next hour. Thus, over a three-hour period in a non-progressive second stage of labour it should become obvious whether there is adequate progress to continue, or cephalopelvic disproportion has become manifest and delivery should be by caesarean section. In the multiparous patient these times should be reduced.

Assessment of progress

Accurate assessment of the level of the fetal head in the pelvis is the essential element of progress in the second stage. This can be quite difficult because of the variables of moulding and caput formation of the fetal head (see Chapter 1). The assessment of moulding and caput is subjective and it can be difficult on vaginal examination alone to accurately assess the true level of the fetal head in relation to the ischial spines. Therefore, a combination of both vaginal and abdominal assessment is necessary to obtain the full picture. The abdominal examination describes the level of the fetal head in fifths above the pelvic brim. One fifth being roughly equal to one fingerbreadth above the pubic symphysis (Notelovitz 1972). A head that is one-fifth palpable above the pelvic brim will be just at the ischial spines. A head that is at spines +1 cm to +2 cm will not be palpable at the pelvic brim.

Maternal position

Throughout the ages women have adopted, or been advised to adopt, just about every position imaginable in the second stage of labour. The general principles of common sense and the woman's own choice should guide matters. The worst position is supine, which is mechanically illogical and also associated with potential aortocaval compression leading to more fetal heart rate abnormalities and lower Apgar scores (DeJong *et al.* 1997). In general, upright positions are more comfortable and logical. Kneeling, squatting, sitting and being on all fours all have their advocates. Some of these positions are quite hard to maintain for long periods of time. It is probably advantageous for the woman to change her position during the second stage of labour and many will choose the semi-recumbent position alternating with squatting, kneeling or the lateral position.

Maternal effort

Maternal bearing-down should not be encouraged until the fetal head has descended to the pelvic floor. This is particularly relevant in the nulliparous woman, in whom full cervical dilatation is often reached when the head is still at the level of the mid pelvis ((Vause *et al.* 1998). At this point, maternal pushing will be unproductive, exhausting and demoralising. There is a limit to how long a woman can push productively in the second stage (usually about one hour) and this resource should not be squandered when the head is at the level of the mid pelvis. The traditional 'coached' method of pushing is to encourage the woman to take a deep breath and push against a closed glottis (Valsalva manoeuvre) for as long as she can hold her breath

– usually about 8–10 seconds. This type of coached pushing is associated with a reduction in the duration of the second stage. However, it is also associated with a rise in maternal intrathoracic pressure, decreased venous return and cardiac output, which can result in reduced uteroplacental circulation. As a result there are more abnormalities of the fetal heart rate, lower cord pH and lower Apgar scores with this technique (Barnett and Humerick 1982). If the woman is not coached she will tend to push for four to six seconds every ten seconds or so during the contraction. Furthermore, she will tend not to use the full Valsalva manoeuvre. The net result is a slightly longer second stage of labour but less disruption to the uteroplacental circulation and therefore better fetal oxygenation.

Changes in fetal heart rate

In normal labour, the fetal heart rate can be monitored adequately by auscultation after each contraction in the second stage. If there is doubt, and in high-risk pregnancies, continuous monitoring of the fetal heart should be carried out because this is the time of maximal hypoxic stress. Details of fetal assessment in labour are covered in Chapter 3. In essence, it is common to see early decelerations in the second stage of labour due to head compression. If there are no other abnormalities these are regarded as physiological. Mild to moderate variable decelerations are also common in the second stage of labour and provided that the recovery is rapid and the baseline variability normal, these need not be a cause for intervention (Kreb 1997).

Analgesia

This may just be an extension of epidural analgesia from the first stage of labour, in which case the previous comments about oxytocin augmentation of the second stage may be relevant. If the patient has not required epidural analgesia, inhalation analgesia – nitrous oxide 50% oxygen 50% – may be effective, particularly for the multiparous woman with a short second stage of labour. Skilful application of this technique is necessary if it is to be beneficial, as outlined in Chapter 1.

If an episiotomy is deemed necessary, infiltration of the perineum with local anaesthetic is appropriate. Analgesic techniques for assisted vaginal delivery are considered in Chapter 7.

Care of the perineum

Every effort should be made to deliver the fetal head over an intact perineum (Kreb 1997). Episiotomy will be required if it is necessary to accelerate delivery for fetal distress and/or the perineum is acting as an obstruction. It may also be required in assisted vaginal delivery if more than a second-degree tear of the perineum is likely to occur. Midline episiotomy is easier to repair and associated with less postoperative pain than a mediolateral episiotomy. However, the midline episiotomy is more likely to extend into the anal sphincter and, for this reason, when episiotomy is indicated a mediolateral type is often performed.

Lacerations and episiotomy should be repaired in layers with careful approximation of the deep muscular levels. If the deeper layers of sutures approximate the skin to within 0.5 cm with the woman in the lithotomy position then skin sutures are not required. If not, a subcuticular stitch is preferable to interrupted skin sutures. Studies have shown that polyfilament sutures are slightly superior to catgut (Mackrodt *et al.* 1998; Renfrew *et al.* 1998).

Third-degree (anal sphincter) and fourth-degree (anal sphincter and rectal mucosa) tears require careful suturing. Long-acting absorbable sutures such as polydioxanone may give a better long-term result than short-term absorbable sutures such as catgut or polyglactin. Whether end-to-end repair of a torn anal sphincter is as good as the overlapping technique has yet to be proven (RCOG 2001). Whichever technique is used the results will be better if a careful repair with adequate anaesthesia and assistance is performed.

While there is an increasing amount of evidence-based data on the second stage of labour much of the management remains *secundum artem*. It is the most dramatic stage of pregnancy when the very essence of the art of midwifery and obstetrics is brought to bear. It is easy for attendants to get caught up in the drama and one therefore has to remember the essential elements, which are the condition of the mother and the fetus, so that hasty ill-considered decisions are not taken which might jeopardise the safety of either.

References

Barnett M, Humerick S. (1982) Infant outcome in relation to second stage of labour pushing method. *Birth* 9:221–9.

Bates RG, Helm CW, Duncan A. (1985) Uterine activity in the second stage of labour and the effect of epidural analgesia. *Br J Obstet Gynaecol* 92:1246–50.

Confidential Inquiry into Stillbirths and Deaths in Infancy. (1997) *4th Annual Report*. London: Maternal and Child Health Research Consortium.

DeJong PR, Johanson RB, Baxen P, Adrians PD, Van der Westhuisen S, Jones PW. (1997) Randomised trial comparing the upright and supine positions for the second stage of labour. *Br J Obstet Gynaecol* 104:567–71.

Goodfellow CF, Howell MGR, Swaab DF. (1983) Oxytocin deficiency at delivery with epidural analgesia. *Br J Obstet Gynaecol* 92:14–19.

Hansen SL, Clark SL, Foster JC. (2002) Active pushing versus passive fetal descent in the second stage: a randomized controlled trial. *Obstet Gynecol* 99:29–34.

Kreb HB. (1997) Intrapartum fetal heart rate monitoring. *Am J Obstet Gynecol* 133:762–80.

Mackrodt C, Gordon B, Fern E, Ayers S, Trusdale A, Grant A. (1998) The Ipswich childbirth study: 2. A randomized comparison of polyglactin 910 with chromic catgut for postpartum perineal repair. *Br J Obstet Gynaecol* 105:41–5.

Menticoglou SM, Manning FA, Harmon CR. (1995) Perinatal outcome in relation to second stage duration. *Am J Obstet Gynecol* 173:906–12.

Notelovitz M. (1972) The graphic monitoring of labour. *S Afr J Obstet Gynaecol* 47:3–7.

Renfrew MJ, Hannah W, Albers L. (1998) Practices that minimize trauma to the genital tract in childbirth: a systematic review of the literature. *Birth* 25:143–6.

Saunders N, Spiby H, Gilvert L. (1989) Oxytocin infusion during second stage of labour in primiparous women using epidural analgesia: A randomised double-blind placebo controlled trial. *BMJ* 299:1423–6.

Vause S, Congdon HM, Thornton J. (1998) Immediate and delayed pushing in the second stage of labour for nulliparous women with epidural analgesia. A randomised controlled trial. *Br J Obstet Gynaecol* 105:186–8.

RCOG. (2001) *Management of Third- and Fourth-degree Perineal Tears Following Vaginal Delivery. Guideline No. 29*. London: Royal College of Obstetricians and Gynaecologists.

3 Fetal surveillance in labour

The Fourth Confidential Inquiry into Stillbirths and Deaths in Infancy (1997) highlighted the need for good fetal surveillance in labour. Suboptimal interpretation of intrapartum fetal heart rate recording, inappropriate action and poor communication were highlighted. Hypoxic brain damage or death of the fetus accounted for almost 40% of the medico-legal claims in the UK. Although hypoxic brain damage was thought to be the cause of 10% of cerebral palsy, recent studies on cerebral palsy attribute 25–30% to intrapartum events in term pregnancies (Hagberg *et al.* 2001).

Fetal heart rate monitoring

The guidelines produced by the National Institute of Clinical Excellence and the Royal College of Obstetricians and Gynaecologists (2001) recommend that those at low risk can be monitored by intermittent auscultation. This entails auscultation of the fetal heart for one minute through a uterine contraction every 15 minutes during the first stage of labour and after every other contraction, or every five minutes, in the second stage of labour. If auscultation shows changes in the baseline rate, decelerations, irregular heart rate, or if there is difficulty with auscultation, continuous electronic fetal heart rate monitoring (EFM) should be undertaken. Continuous cardiotocography (CTG) should be used for all labours with high risk factors shown in Table 3.1.

A screening admission test with CTG has been proposed and used in many hospitals (Ingemarsson *et al.* 1986). If this is completely normal and the subsequent progress of labour is appropriate, then the risk of fetal hypoxia developing is rare and intermittent auscultation can be used. However, the RCOG guidelines do not recommend an admission CTG in low risk labour. A variation on this theme has been a study using Doppler ultrasound to enhance the usual auscultation with a fetal stethoscope (Mires *et al.* 2001). Ironically, this 'low-tech' intermittent auscultation requires more stringent one-to-one nursing care in labour, which is the ideal. However, staffing limitations sometimes dictate that continuous CTG is offered instead.

Table 3.1 Indications for continuous cardiotocography (RCOG 2001)

Indication	*Risk factor*
Antepartum	Previous caesarean section Pre-eclampsia Post-term pregnancy (> 42 weeks) Prolonged membrane rupture (> 24 hours) Diabetes Induced labour Antepartum haemorrhage Other maternal medical disease
Fetal	Growth restriction Prematurity Oligohydramnios Abnormal Doppler artery velocimetry Multiple pregnancies Meconium-stained liquor Breech presentation
Intrapartum	Oxytocin augmentation Epidural analgesia Vaginal bleeding in labour Maternal pyrexia Fresh meconium stained liquor

CARDIOTOCOGRAPHY: BASIC CONSIDERATIONS AND FETAL HEART RATE PATTERNS

The FHR tracing has four recognisable features: baseline rate, baseline variability, accelerations and decelerations (Ingemarsson *et al.* 1993; Gibb and Arulkumaran 1997). A classification of CTG traces is given in Table 3.2.

Baseline rate

The baseline rate is calculated by drawing a line through the variability of the trace where there are no accelerations or decelerations. The normal baseline rate at term is 110–160 bpm (RCOG 2001).

Baseline variability

Baseline variability represents the integrity of the autonomic nervous system (sympathetic and parasympathetic) and is the bandwidth of the up and down excursions or 'wiggliness' of the trace. Normal baseline variability is 5–25 bpm. Reduced baseline variability is less than 5 bpm and the CTG is considered suspicious if it is reduced for longer than 40 minutes but less than 90 minutes, and abnormal if reduced for longer than 90 minutes (RCOG 2001).

Table 3.2 Classification of the cardiotocograph (CTG) and intrapartum trace (RCOG 2001)	
Classification	*Definition*
Cardiotocograph	
Normal	All four features fall into the category
Suspicious	A CTG whose features fall into one of the non-reassuring categories and the remainder of the features are reassuring
Pathological	A CTG whose features fall into two or more non-reassuring categories or one or more abnormal categories
Intrapartum trace	
Reassuring	Baseline rate 110–160 bpm Baseline variability > 5 bpm, 2 accelerations in 20 minutes and no decelerations
Non-reassuring	Abnormal baseline rate 100–109 bpm or 161–180 bpm; reduced baseline variability, < 5 bpm for > 40 minutes but < 90 minutes; early deceleration; variable deceleration, single prolonged deceleration up to 3 minutes
Abnormal	Abnormal baseline rate < 100, > 180, sinusoidal pattern for > 10 minutes; variability < 5 bpm for equal or greater than 90 minutes Late decelerations, atypical variable decelerations (with ominous features duration > 60 seconds, beat loss > 60 bpm, late recovery, late deceleration component, poor baseline variability between and/or during decelerations); single prolonged deceleration > 3 minutes

Accelerations

An acceleration is an abrupt rise in the baseline rate by more than 15 beats lasting for longer than 15 seconds from onset to end. They are usually associated with fetal movements or other fetal stimulation by uterine contractions or during a pelvic examination. A functioning somatic nervous system and brain stem centres are necessary for fetal movements and associated accelerations. Accelerations and normal baseline variability are hallmarks of normal fetal oxygenation (Figure 3.1).

Decelerations

Decelerations are a drop in the baseline rate of more than 15 beats for longer than 15 seconds. Decelerations that last less than 30 seconds and immediately follow an acceleration are normal reflex changes in the fetal heart rate.

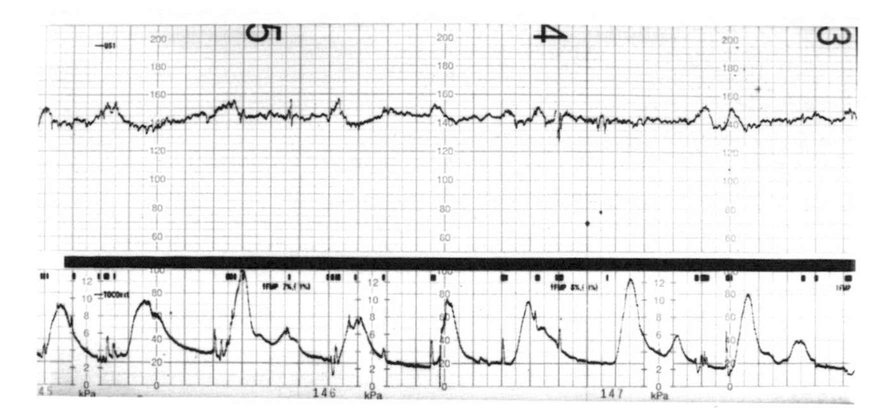

Figure 3.1 A fetal heart rate trace showing features of normal baseline rate, normal baseline variability and accelerations; an active period with accelerations and good baseline variability alternates with a quiet period with reduced baseline variability and no accelerations in a healthy fetus

The placenta acts as the respiratory organ of the fetus *in utero* for gas exchange. Disturbance of fetoplacental circulation by compression of the umbilical cord or a reduction in uteroplacental circulation can cause hypoxia and acidosis in the fetus.

When the umbilical cord gets compressed, the thin-walled vein is occluded first, while blood from the fetus still leaves via the unoccluded arteries. The resultant hypotension causes a slight increase in the fetal heart rate. However, the umbilical arteries are also soon constricted, which causes relative hypertension leading to a sudden fall in the heart rate mediated by the baroreceptor mechanism. Once the pressure is

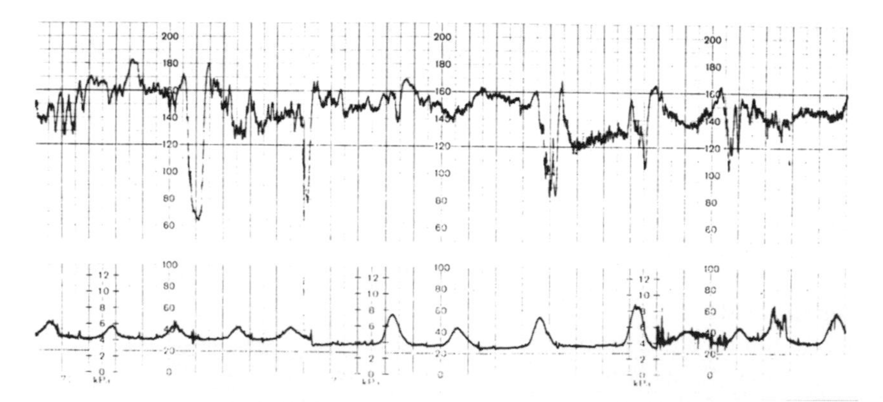

Figure 3.2 A fetal heart rate trace showing variable decelerations

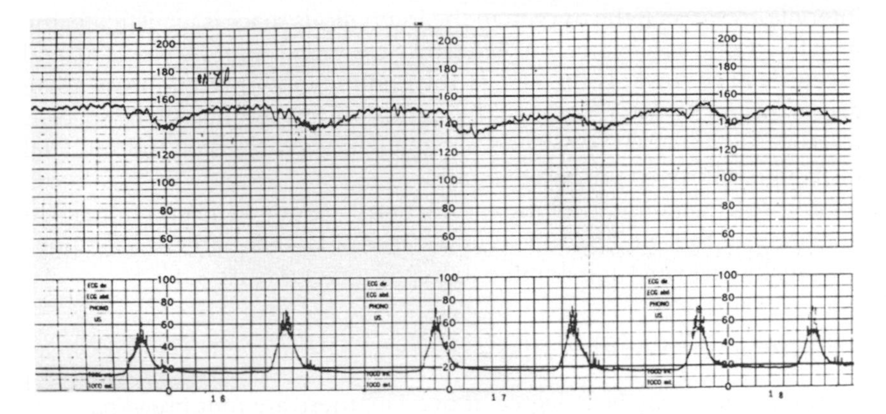

Figure 3.3 A fetal heart rate trace showing late accelerations

released, the artery, due to its thicker wall, opens first and the fetus pumps blood away from the body causing a relative hypotension that results in a slight rise in the heart rate above baseline. This results in the characteristic post-deceleration hump of the variable deceleration (Figure 3.2). As the uterine contraction abates, the pressure on the cord is reduced further, the vein opens and perfusion to and from the fetus is re-established and the fetal heart rate returns to normal.

During a uterine contraction there is cessation of blood flow into the uterus but the fetus continues to receive oxygen from the blood in the

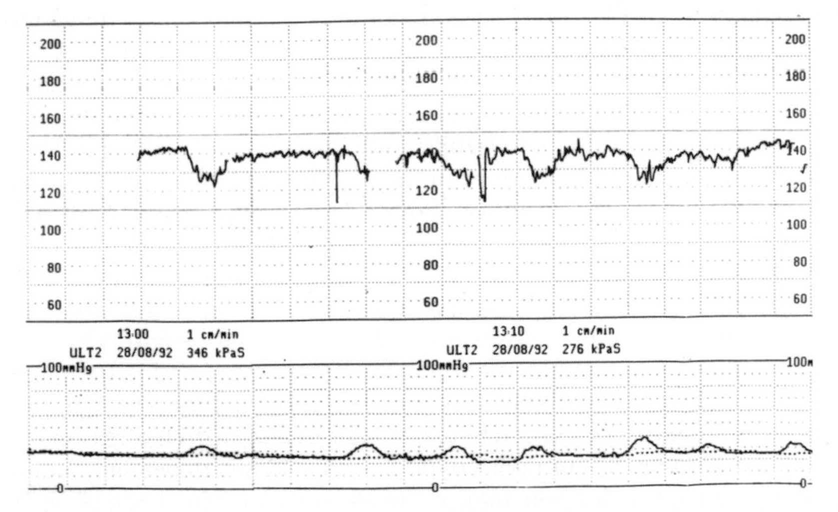

Figure 3.4 A fetal heart rate trace showing early decelerations

intervillous space. If the oxygen in the intervillous space is inadequate, the fetal heart rate decelerates, mediated by a chemoreceptor mechanism, and this is delayed towards the end of the contraction – presenting as a late deceleration (Figure 3.3). Once the perfusion to the intervillous space is re-established, the fetus receives adequate oxygen transfer and the fetal heart rate returns to the baseline rate.

Early decelerations mirror the contractions, are due to head compression and occur in the late first and second stages of labour. Early decelerations are vagally mediated and not due to hypoxaemia (Figure 3.4).

Patterns of fetal hypoxia

Although there may be a degree of overlap, there are four broad patterns of fetal hypoxia that may present during labour.

GRADUALLY DEVELOPING HYPOXIA

Hypoxia can develop gradually, due to repeated occlusion of the umbilical cord, manifest by variable decelerations or due to decreased perfusion to the retroplacental intervillous space reducing the oxygen exchange during contractions, manifest by late decelerations. Hypoxia is unlikely to develop during labour without fetal heart rate decelerations unless hypoxia already exists or some other pathology inhibits this response. Decelerations in the absence of a rise in the baseline rate or reduction in baseline variability indicates the presence of stress due to cord compression or reduced uteroplacental perfusion. With repeated frequent decelerations, one of the first signs that indicate developing fetal hypoxia is the cessation of accelerations. The fetus responds to hypoxia by increasing the cardiac output and increasing the heart rate to circulate more blood through the placenta in an effort to get more oxygen, as it does not have the capacity to significantly increase stroke volume. Thus, with increasing hypoxia there is an increase in the baseline rate until it reaches a plateau. This period is considered to be a 'stress-to-distress interval'. In parallel with this baseline tachycardia there is a gradual reduction in the baseline variability. This combination of a stable tachycardia with silent or flat baseline variability is a sign that the autonomic system of the fetus is probably hypoxaemic (Figure 3.5). This is sometimes referred to as the 'distress period'. With this pattern, the progress of hypoxia and acidosis cannot be predicted by observing the fetal heart pattern alone. If there is not intervention within a reasonable time the fetus may be born with hypoxia and acidosis. Depending on the clinical situation a decision may be made for fetal blood sampling or delivery at this stage. If the situation is ignored, the fetal heart rate can

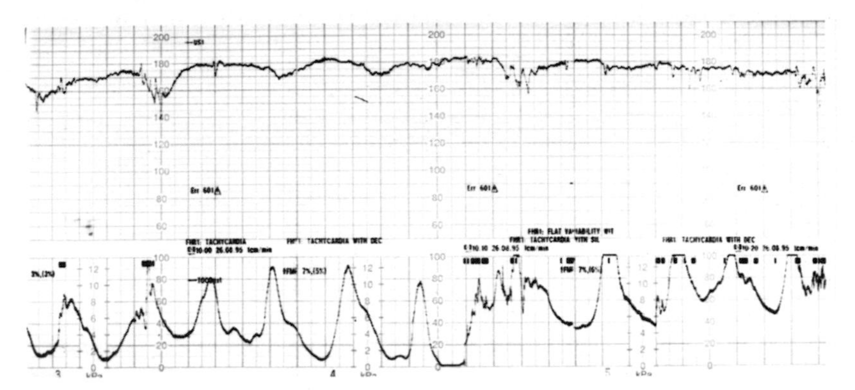

Figure 3.5 A fetal heart rate trace showing the distress period

decline rapidly in a stepwise manner leading to terminal bradycardia. This period is termed the 'distress-to-death interval' and can be quite short (20–60 minutes).

CHRONIC HYPOXIA

A fetus with chronic, pre-existing hypoxia before the onset of labour may show a non-reactive trace with a silent or absent baseline variability, together with shallow decelerations of less than 15 bpm, which may start with the onset of uterine contractions but not recover until after the contraction is over. Although the traditional definition of a deceleration is a drop in the baseline of more than 15 beats for longer than 15 seconds, this combination of shallow decelerations with absent baseline variability is the most ominous of all fetal heart rate tracings. These chronically hypoxic fetuses may have a normal baseline heart rate (110–160 bpm) or a mild tachycardia (Figure 3.6). This is the most consistently ominous pattern and these fetuses can deteriorate and die within a short time. With the stress of uterine contractions, early delivery is indicated.

ACUTE HYPOXIA

Acute accidents such as placental abruption, uterine rupture and scar dehiscence, or cord prolapse, may present with prolonged bradycardia. Other reversible causes of prolonged bradycardia are epidural analgesia and uterine hyperstimulation. Hypoxia and acidosis are likely to result if bradycardia continues for more than ten minutes. Fetal death or neonatal hypoxic sequelae may occur if action is not taken. Those fetuses with clinical signs of placental abruption, uterine rupture or cord prolapse require immediate delivery. In the absence of such an obvious cause,

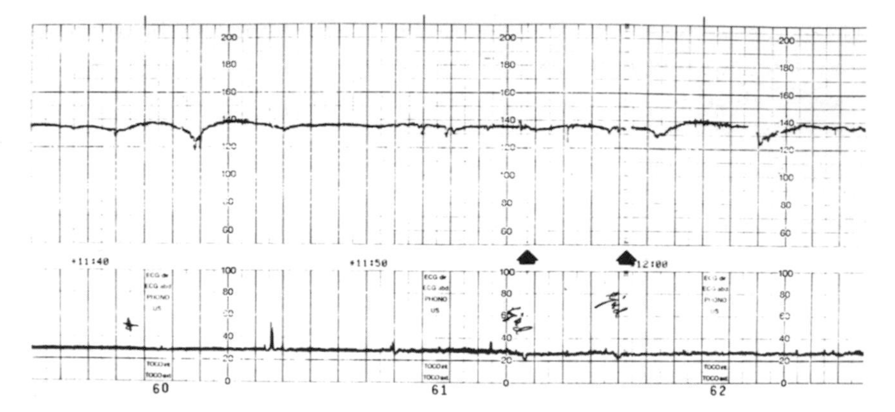

Figure 3.6 A fetal heart rate trace showing reduced variability and shallow decelerations

simple measures include repositioning the woman to relieve presumed cord entanglement and stopping any oxytocin infusion. If the bradycardia is due to uterine hyperstimulation, most often following prostaglandin administration, then acute tocolysis such as terbutaline 0.25 mg subcutaneously or intravenously in 5 ml saline over five minutes may alleviate the situation (Ingemarsson *et al.* 1985a,b).

SUBACUTE HYPOXIA

Profound decelerations of more than 60 beats from the baseline and falling to less than 80 bpm and prolonged for over 90 seconds and recovery to the baseline for periods of less than 30 seconds can cause hypoxia and acidosis

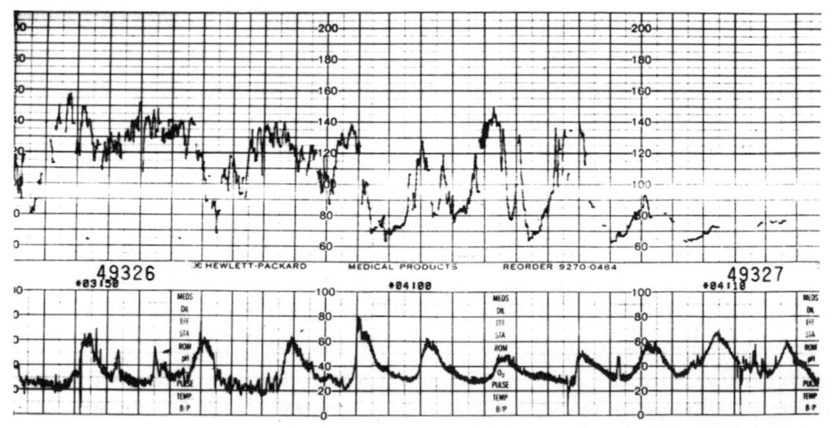

Figure 3.7 A fetal heart rate trace showing prolonged decelerations followed by bradycardia

within one or two hours. With this pattern, the baseline fetal heart rate is normal for a much shorter period compared with the time it is below the baseline rate. Thus, the amount of circulation through the placenta to bring about gas exchange is markedly reduced causing rapid accumulation of carbon dioxide and respiratory acidosis in the fetal circulation, followed by anaerobic metabolism and metabolic acidosis due to inadequate oxygen transfer. With such a trace the baseline heart rate does not rise but there may be a terminal bradycardia (Figure 3.7).

IMPORTANT POINTS TO CONSIDER WHILE INTERPRETING A FETAL HEART RATE TRACE

- Accelerations and normal baseline variability are hallmarks of fetal health.
- Accelerations with reduced baseline variability should be considered suspicious.
- Periods of decreased variability may represent fetal sleep.
- Hypoxic fetuses may have a normal baseline FHR of 110–160 bpm with no accelerations and baseline variability of < 5 bpm for > 40 minutes.
- With baseline variability < 5 bpm even shallow decelerations < 15 bpm are ominous in a non-reactive tracing.
- Placental abruption, cord prolapse and scar rupture can give rise to acute hypoxia and should be identified clinically.
- Hypoxia and acidosis may develop faster with an abnormal trace in patients with scanty thick meconium, intrauterine growth restriction, intrauterine infection with pyrexia, and those who are pre- or post-term.
- In preterm (especially at less than 34 weeks of gestation), hypoxia and acidosis can predispose to hyaline membrane disease, respiratory distress syndrome and may contribute to intraventricular haemorrhage and sequelae warranting early action in the presence of an abnormal trace.
- Injudicious use of oxytocin, epidural anaesthesia and difficult deliveries can worsen hypoxia.
- During labour, if decelerations are absent, asphyxia is unlikely but cannot be excluded.
- Abnormal patterns may represent effects of drugs, fetal anomaly, infection, cerebral haemorrhage and not only hypoxia.

Fetal blood sampling

The clinical risk status, parity of the woman, the stage and rate of progress of labour and the evolving fetal heart rate pattern should determine the need for fetal blood sampling (FBS). It may be of special benefit in those fetuses that are more prone to acidosis, such as those with intrauterine growth restriction, those who are post-term and those with thick meconium and oligohydramnios. Other factors in labour that have a significant influence on the rate of decline of pH are the use of oxytocin, difficult instrumental delivery and acute events such as cord prolapse, uterine scar rupture or placental abruption. In the latter clinical situations, the fetal heart rate pattern can become ominous in a short time and FBS is not helpful as immediate delivery is required. When abnormalities of the baseline rate and variability start to appear, and particularly if the progress of labour is satisfactory, FBS and determination of the fetal pH will help to confirm or deny whether labour should be allowed to continue to progress towards vaginal delivery. In the presence of normal baseline variability and fetal heart accelerations, hypoxia and acidosis are extremely unlikely.

FBS is performed with the mother in the left lateral position to avoid aortocaval compression. Contraindications include fetal bleeding disorders, prematurity (less than 34 weeks of gestation) and maternal infection such as hepatitis, HIV, and herpes. FBS is carried out if other remedial measures, such as intravenous hydration, stopping oxytocin infusion, altering maternal position and tocolytics, if required to correct hyperstimulation, have failed. If the FBS shows the pH to be greater than 7.25 it can be repeated in 30–60 minutes in the presence of continued fetal heart rate abnormality. Over this period, the rate of progress of labour and the decline in pH between the two samples, together with the clinical context should guide the subsequent management of labour. If the pH is between 7.21 and 7.24 the sample should be repeated within 30 minutes and a further decline and/or a deterioration in the FHR pattern and clinical picture, may warrant immediate delivery. If the pH is less than 7.20, delivery is indicated.

Meta-analysis of trials shows that intrapartum EFM without supporting FBS is associated with a significant increase in delivery by caesarean section with no apparent benefit in neonatal outcome.

Additional tests of fetal surveillance

STIMULATION TESTS

Acceleration of the fetal heart in response to the stimulus of FBS lead to the observation that in such cases fetal acidosis almost never occurred.

Thus, was developed the fetal scalp stimulation test (Elimian *et al.*1997; Skupski *et al.* 2002). This can be performed using Allis or similar forceps to pinch the fetal scalp. Accelerations of greater than 15 bpm and longer than 15 seconds almost exclude fetal acidosis. A similar response has been found to a vibroacoustic stimulus (Edershiem *et al.* 1987), which is non-invasive and further research in this area has been recommended (RCOG 2001).

FETAL ELECTROCARDIOGRAM WAVEFORM ANALYSIS AND PULSE OXIMETRY

Published studies show that analysis of fetal electrocardiogram (ECG) waveforms may be a useful adjunct to CTG, leading to both a reduction in the caesarean section rate and the incidence of metabolic acidosis of the newborn.

Continuous fetal oxygen saturation monitoring with pulse oximeter may provide additional information and may be useful in evaluating the association of hypoxia with abnormal fetal heart rate patterns. However, randomised trials have failed to show an overall reduction in the operative delivery rate.

AMNIOINFUSION

This simple technique has been shown to reduce the persistence of certain abnormal fetal heart rate patterns (variable and prolonged decelerations) and decrease the caesarean section rate for 'fetal distress' (Mizazaki and Nevarez 1985). It may also reduce the morbidity and sequelae of meconium aspiration in the neonate (Mohomed *et al.* 1998). Warmed physiological saline is infused via a transcervical catheter at a rate of approximately 15 ml/minute, i.e. about 500 ml in 30 minutes.

SUMMARY

It is common for fetal heart rate changes to occur due to factors other than hypoxia. Maternal dehydration, ketosis, pyrexia and anxiety can cause fetal tachycardia. Oxytocin can lead to hyperstimulation and late decelerations. Prolonged bradycardia may follow hypotension due to postural changes or after epidural analgesia. Thus, when fetal heart rate changes occur ,one should correlate the changes with the clinical picture and take rational action. In many instances, remedial action such as maternal rehydration, repositioning the mother, stopping oxytocin infusion or amnioinfusion will restore the fetal heart rate to normal. At the other extreme, acute clinical events such as cord prolapse, uterine scar rupture or placental abruption will dictate immediate delivery of the fetus. In cases between these two extremes, the presence of meconium, quantity of amniotic fluid, stage and rate of progress of labour, as well as the characteristics of the fetal heart rate tracing will guide management. Fetal scalp stimulation is a simple and useful adjunct to heart rate interpretation. If the abnormal fetal heart rate persists, FBS may be appropriate. The newer tests of fetal ECG waveform analysis and pulse oximetry have been shown to be useful and their role in clinical management should be clarified in the near future.

References

Confidential Inquiry into Stillbirths and Deaths in Infancy. (1997) *4th Annual Report 1995*. London: Maternal and Child Health Research Consortium.

Edersheim TG, Hutson JM, Druzin ML, Kogut EA. (1987) Fetal heart response to vibratory acoustic stimulation predicts pH in labour. *Am J Obstet Gynecol* 157:1557–60.

Elimian A, Figueroa R, Tejani N. (1997) Intrapartum assessment of fetal well-being: a comparison of scalp stimulation with scalp blood pH sampling. *Obstet Gynecol* 89:373–6.

Gibb DMF, Arulkumaran S. (1997) *Fetal Monitoring in Practice*. 2nd ed. London: Butterworth Heinemann.

Hagberg B, Hagberg G, Beckung E, Uvebrant P. (2001) Changing panorama of cerebral palsy in Sweden. VII. Prevalence and origin in the birth year period 1991–1994. *Acta Paediatr* 90:271–7.

Ingemarsson I. Arulkumaran S, Ratnam SS. (1985a) Single injection of terbutaline in term labour I. Effect of fetal pH in cases with prolonged bradycardia. *Am J Obstet Gynecol* 153:859–65.

Ingemarsson I. Arulkumaran S, Ratnam SS. (1985b) Single injection of terbutaline in term labour II. Effect on uterine activity. *Am J Obstet Gynecol* 153:865–9.

Ingemarsson I, Arulkumaran S, Ingemarsson E, Tambryraja RL, Ratnam SS. (1986) Admission test: a screening test for fetal distress in labor. *Obstet Gynecol* 68:800–6.

Ingemarsson I, Ingemarsson E, Spencer JAD. (1993) *Practical Guide to Fetal Heart Rate Monitoring*. Oxford: Oxford University Press.

Mires G, Williams F, Howie P. (2001) Randomised controlled trial of cardiotocography versus Doppler auscultation of fetal heart at admission in labour in low risk obstetric population. *BMJ* 322:1457–62.

Mizazaki FS, Nevarez F. (1985) Saline amniotic infusion for relief of repetitive variable decelerations: a prospective randomized study. *Am J Obstet Gynecol* 153:301–3.

Mahomed K, Mulambo T, Woelk G, Hofmeyr GJ, Gulmezoglu AM. (1998) The Collaborative Randomised Amnioinfusion for Meconium Project (CRAMP): Zimbabwe. *Br J Obstet Gynaecol* 105:309–13.

Rathmore AM, Singh R, Ramji S, Tripathi R. (2002) Randomised trial of amnioinfusion during labour with meconium stained amniotic fluid. *Br J Obstet*

Gynaecol 109:17–20.

Royal College of Obstetricians and Gynaecologists. (2001) *The Use of Electronic Fetal Monitoring. Evidence-based Clinical Guidelines No. 8*. London: RCOG Press.

Skupski DW, Rosenberg CR, Eglinton GS. (2002) Intrapartum fetal stimulation tests: a meta-analysis. *Obstet Gynecol* 99:129–34.

4 Third stage of labour

The third stage of labour lasts from the birth of the infant until delivery of the placenta. It usually lasts 5–10 minutes and rarely more than 30 minutes. Although it is the shortest of the three stages of labour, it carries the most potential risk for the mother.

Physiology

After delivery of the infant, the uterus continues to contract rhythmically. The muscle fibres of the uterus, which have stretched considerably to accommodate the fetus, are shortened dramatically by these contractions and sustained by retraction. Retraction is that property, unique to the uterus by which the muscle fibre length is permanently shortened after the active, energy-consuming contraction has passed.

PLACENTAL SEPARATION

Contraction and retraction of the uterine muscle causes a progressive reduction in the size of the placental implantation site. Thus, the relatively inelastic placenta buckles and is sheared from the uterine wall. An additional, but much less significant, role involves compression of the decidual veins by the uterine contraction, while the spiral arteries continue to pump blood into the intervillous space. This extravasation of blood helps dissect through the decidua spongiosa layer. Once the placenta has physically separated from the uterine wall the contractions assist its passage from the uterine cavity, through the cervix and into the upper vagina.

HAEMOSTASIS

Separation of the placenta leaves a vascular placental bed with torn blood vessels. However, the uterine muscle fibres are arranged in a criss-cross fashion and the vessels pass through this latticework. As a result, when the uterine muscle contracts the vessels are effectively compressed by these physiological sutures or living ligatures. This anatomical and physiological mechanism is one of the haemostatic marvels of the human body.

SIGNS OF PLACENTAL SEPARATION

1. The uterine fundus rises and changes from a broad discoid shape to a more narrow globular form due to the placenta separating and leaving the upper uterine segment.
2. As the edge of the placenta separates from the uterine wall bleeding will occur – usually a fairly brisk gush of blood. This is not a completely reliable sign as bleeding may start when only part of the placenta has separated or, conversely, may not be seen at all when the entire placenta has separated but the blood is contained behind the membranes.
3. Cord lengthening of 8–15 cm is the most reliable sign.

Management

After delivery of the infant, the cord is clamped, divided and appropriate cord blood samples are collected. The woman is then closely observed for signs of placental separation. While waiting for these signs, the attendant places the cord clamp at the level of the introitus so that cord lengthening can be appreciated. One hand should cradle and guard the fundus in order to appreciate the uterine signs of placental separation or, alternatively, aid early detection of an atonic uterus filling with blood. The uterine hand should not manipulate the fundus as this interference may increase blood loss or stimulate a constriction ring causing retained placenta. When the clinical signs of separation occur, the attendant delivers the placenta by controlled cord traction. For this manoeuvre, one hand is placed on the lower part of the uterus just above the symphysis and presses gently upwards and backwards as steady traction with the other hand on the clamp delivers the placenta (Figure 4.1). The placenta is then carefully examined to ensure it is complete.

There are two approaches to the routine management of the third stage of labour: expectant or physiological and active.

EXPECTANT OR PHYSIOLOGICAL MANAGEMENT

In essence, this technique is to await the normal physiological changes that bring about placental separation and haemostasis. This approach is favoured by women and their attendants who prefer limited intervention in the management of labour. Immediate suckling after birth is encouraged in order to reduce blood loss and postpartum haemorrhage (Chua *et al.* 1994). Unfortunately, this physiologically attractive approach was found not to be effective in a randomised trial (Bullough *et al.* 1989).

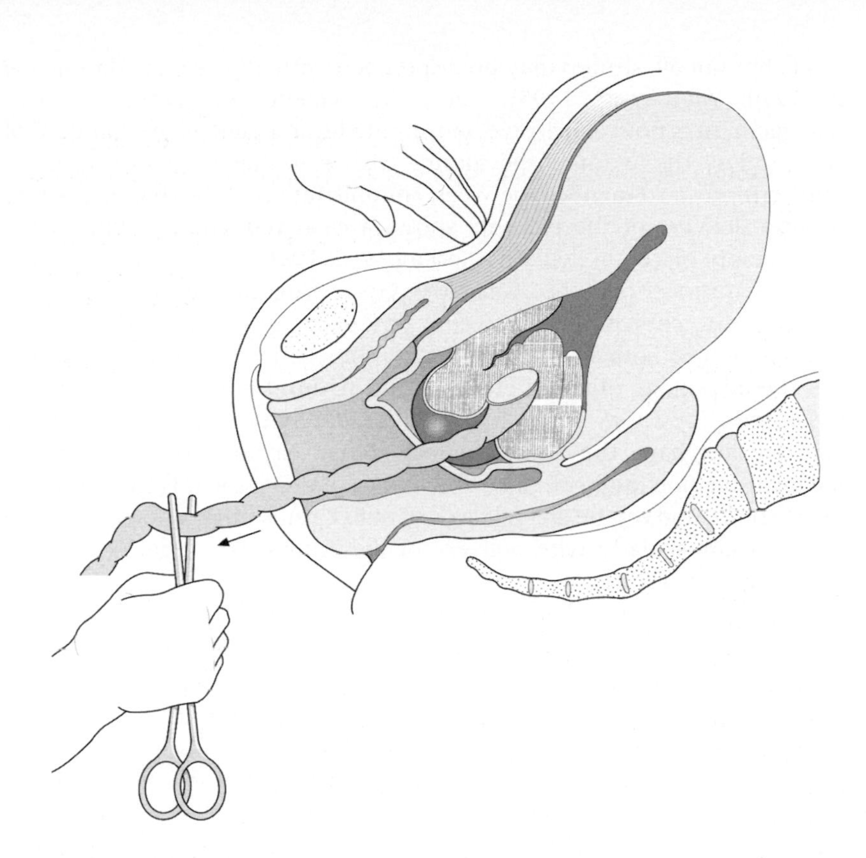

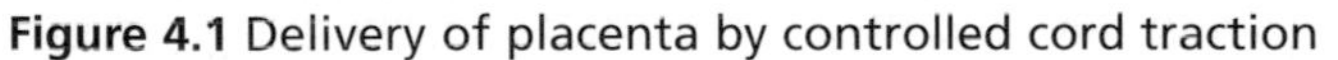
Figure 4.1 Delivery of placenta by controlled cord traction

ACTIVE MANAGEMENT

This involves giving an oxytocic drug at or just after delivery of the infant in order to induce an early and consistent uterine contraction, thereby producing placental separation and haemostasis without delay. Postpartum haemorrhage (PPH) is dealt with in Chapter 16, but routine active management of the third stage of labour is aimed at preventing this, the most common complication of the third stage. Randomised controlled trials have consistently shown that blood loss, PPH and the need for blood transfusion are all reduced by 40–50% when active is compared with expectant management (Prendiville *et al.* 1988; Nordstrom *et al.* 1997; Rogers *et al.* 1998). Active management using oxytocin does not increase the risk of retained placenta, nor does it increase nausea and vomiting. Ergometrine does increase the incidence of nausea and vomiting and in some, but not all, studies may predispose to retained placenta (Hammar *et al.* 1990; Yuen *et al.* 1995). Thus, the evidence in favour of active management is now conclusive and should be accepted as the standard of care, unless the woman specifically wishes to have no intervention. Furthermore, a comparison between administration of the oxytocic before or after delivery of the placenta shows a clear reduction in PPH when given before placental delivery (Soriano *et al.* 1996).

The characteristics of the available oxytocic drugs are outlined below. At present the choice lies between oxytocin and ergometrine or a combination of both in the product Syntometrine® (Alliance). Oxytocin has the advantage of being effective and without adverse effects in the dose used (Choy *et al.* 2002). Ergometrine and Syntometrine® are equally effective but have the adverse effect of nausea and vomiting and an inconclusive potential risk of retained placenta. Oxytocin is therefore the safest choice and can be given in a dose of five units intravenously or 5–10 units intramuscularly with delivery of the anterior shoulder or as soon thereafter as feasible.

The woman is also vulnerable to uterine atony and haemorrhage in the first few hours postpartum. Close observation, particularly for the first two to three hours postpartum, is therefore essential. During this time, the uterus should be regularly massaged to ensure that it is well contracted. As a full bladder can interfere with uterine retraction it should be kept empty. If an intravenous drip is already in place then the addition of 20 units oxytocin to 500 ml crystalloid will assist in maintaining uterine contractions. If ergometrine or Syntometrine® has been used, their more prolonged effect usually accomplishes this without further doses. No part of active management of labour need interfere with the new parents' involvement with and attachment to their new baby.

Oxytocic drugs

OXYTOCIN

Oxytocin is the cheapest and safest oxytocic drug. It produces rapid, rhythmic uterine contractions lasting for 15–30 minutes. Oxytocin has transient relaxant effects on vascular smooth muscle. It may produce a mild and clinically insignificant reduction in blood pressure due to reduced total peripheral resistance. The dose is 5 units intravenously, 10 units intramuscularly or via an intravenous infusion such as 20 units in 500 ml crystalloid. Because of its safety and lack of contraindications, oxytocin is the oxytocic drug of first choice. The characteristics of the oxytocic drugs are summarised in Table 4.1.

Table 4.1 Oxytocic drugs

Drug	*Dose and route*	*Duration of action*	*Adverse effects*	*Contraindications*
Oxytocin	5 units IV 10 units IM 20 units in 500 ml infusion	15–30 minutes	Insignificant hypotension and flushing Water intoxication in high doses (> 200 units)	None
Ergometrine	0.2–0.25 mg IV or IM	1–2 hours	Nausea, vomiting Hypertension Vasospasm	Pre-eclampsia/hypertension Cardiovascular disease
Syntometrine® (Alliance) (5 units oxytocin 0.5 mg ergometrine)	1 ampoule IM	1–2 hours	Nausea, vomiting Hypertension Vasospasm	Pre-eclampsia/hypertension Cardiovascular disease
15-methyl PGF2α	0.25 mg IM or IMM 0.25 mg in 500 ml infusion	4–6 hours	Vomiting Diarrhoea Flushing Shivering Pyrexia Vasospasm Bronchospasm	Cardiovascular disease Asthma
Misoprostol	400–600 μg oral	1–2 hours	Nausea Diarrhoea Shivering Pyrexia	None

IM = intramuscular; IMM = intramyometrial; IV = intravenous

ERGOMETRINE

Ergometrine has been used for 65 years and has pride of place in the history of prevention and management of postpartum haemorrhage (Baskett 2000). It induces prolonged uterine contractions for 60–120 minutes. It produces peripheral vasoconstriction, which, in the normal woman, is usually not clinically significant. However, in patients with pre-eclampsia or chronic hypertension, this effect can be pronounced and can precipitate a hypertensive crisis or eclamptic fit. It is therefore contraindicated in all patients with hypertensive disease. Ergometrine-induced vasoconstriction is responsive to intravenous chlorpromazine or glyceryl trinitrate. On very rare occasions, ergometrine can induce coronary artery spasm and isolated cases of myocardial infarction have been attributed to its use. In the context of the millions of women who have received ergometrine such cases are incredibly rare. Coronary artery spasm induced by ergometrine should respond to intravenous glyceryl trinitrate. Nausea and vomiting are also common adverse effects of ergometrine, occurring in up to 20–25% of women. The dose is 0.2–0.25 mg, preferably by intramuscular injection but, if the need is urgent, it can be given intravenously. The higher dose of 0.5 mg should not be given initially as it is associated with increased adverse effects without greater efficacy. Recent trials have indicated that rectal administration in effective.

SYNTOMETRINE®

Syntometrine® is a combination of 5.0 units of oxytocin and 0.5 mg ergometrine and thus combines the rapid onset of oxytocin with the more prolonged effect of ergometrine. It carries the same complications and contraindications as ergometrine, although the mild vasodilatation effect of oxytocin may to some extent ameliorate the vasopressor effect of ergometrine.

15-METHYL PROSTAGLANDIN $F_{2}\alpha$

15-methyl prostaglandin $F_{2}\alpha$ (carboprost; Hemabate®, Pharmacia) has a much stronger uterotonic effect than its parent compound, resulting in good oxytocic action with much less of the undesirable smooth muscle stimulatory effects (vasoconstriction, bronchoconstriction, nausea and vomiting). Flushing, shivering, and pyrexia (37.5–38.5°C) are not uncommon but relatively mild adverse effects. The dose is 0.25 mg intramuscularly or intramyometrially. Most authors agree that an intravenous bolus should be avoided because of the possibility of more profound smooth muscle stimulation adverse effects, although it has been used many times by that route without ill effect. For rapid onset the intramyometrial route is preferred and this is achieved by diluting the 1-ml ampoule containing 0.25 mg in 5 ml physiological saline and injecting this transabdominally with a 20-gauge spinal needle in two sites into the uterine fundus. The duration of action is up to six hours. This drug has proved valuable as a second-line agent in cases of uterine atony unresponsive to oxytocin and ergometrine (Hyashi *et al.* 1984; Oleen and Mariano 1990). 15-methyl prostaglandin $F_{2}\alpha$ can also be given as a dilute solution of 0.25 mg in 500 ml saline and administered as an infusion (Granstrom *et al.* 1989).

MISOPROSTOL

Misoprostol is an analogue of prostaglandin E_1 and is cheap and stable with a prolonged shelf life. It can be given orally, which, together with the properties mentioned above, makes it a potentially attractive option for routine active management of the third stage of labour, particularly in developing countries (El-Refaey *et al.* 1997, 2000; Goldberg *et al.* 2001; Gülmezoglu *et al.* 2001; Kundodiwa *et al.* 2001; Ng *et al.* 2001). The most commonly used oral dose is 400–600 μg. The main adverse effects are shivering, mild pyrexia and diarrhoea.

Retained placenta

With expectant management of the third stage, the placenta is usually delivered within 10–20 minutes. With active management this time is halved. The incidence of retained placenta 30 minutes after delivery of the infant is about 2–4% and at 60 minutes post-delivery it is half of this. The longer the placenta is retained the greater the risk of postpartum haemorrhage. In most cases the treatment is manual removal of the placenta under anaesthesia. Thus, in the absence of active bleeding, the decision as to when to proceed to manual removal depends to a large extent on the availability of safe anaesthesia. If the patient has regional anaesthesia *in situ* for delivery there is little to be gained by waiting longer than 15–20 minutes before proceeding to manual removal. If, however, anaesthesia has to be induced, most will wait for 30 minutes and then marshal the resources to provide anaesthesia. This usually takes 20–30 minutes, so that manual removal is usually done about 60 minutes following delivery of the infant. By waiting 30–60 minutes the placenta will deliver spontaneously in half of these cases (Selinger *et al.* 1986). Obviously, this slower approach to manual removal is only valid if there is no active bleeding. If haemorrhage supervenes then immediate steps to remove the placenta must be taken.

CAUSES OF RETAINED PLACENTA

The placenta that has separated from the uterine wall may be retained due to uterine atony or the presence of a uterine constriction ring.

Retained adherent placenta can be due to ordinary adherence with failure of separation through the decidua spongiosa layer or pathological adherence due to a deficient decidual reaction allowing invasion of the myometrium by the trophoblast. This is more likely in a uterine site previously affected by surgery, trauma or infection.

THE THREE DEGREES OF PATHOLOGICAL ADHERENCE

- Placenta accreta – adherence to the myometrium
- Placenta increta – invading the myometrium
- Placenta percreta – penetrating through the myometrium to the serosal layer.

The placenta that is praevia is more likely to be pathologically adherent because of the poor decidual response of the lower uterine segment. It is rare for the entire placental surface to be pathologically adherent but areas of partial accreta will be encountered.

MANAGEMENT OF RETAINED PLACENTA

If the retained placenta is associated with uterine atony or a constriction ring then haemorrhage is more likely. If so, the haemorrhage is treated with intravenous oxytocin and steps are taken to deliver the placenta. Ultimately, the management of retained placenta is manual removal (Figure 4.2). Timing and anaesthetic considerations have already been discussed.

TECHNIQUE FOR MANUAL REMOVAL OF THE PLACENTA

After induction of suitable anaesthesia, place the well-lubricated right or left hand in the vagina and follow the cord up through the cervix. With the opposite hand, firmly cradle and push down on the uterine fundus.

The fingers and thumb of the uterine hand should be kept extended and used as one unit to find the lower margin of the placenta and, with side-to-side movements, find and separate through the plane of cleavage. Once the placenta has been completely separated, it should be grasped and slowly removed through the cervix. It is important not to do this too rapidly as it is possible to invert the uterus if part of the placenta remains

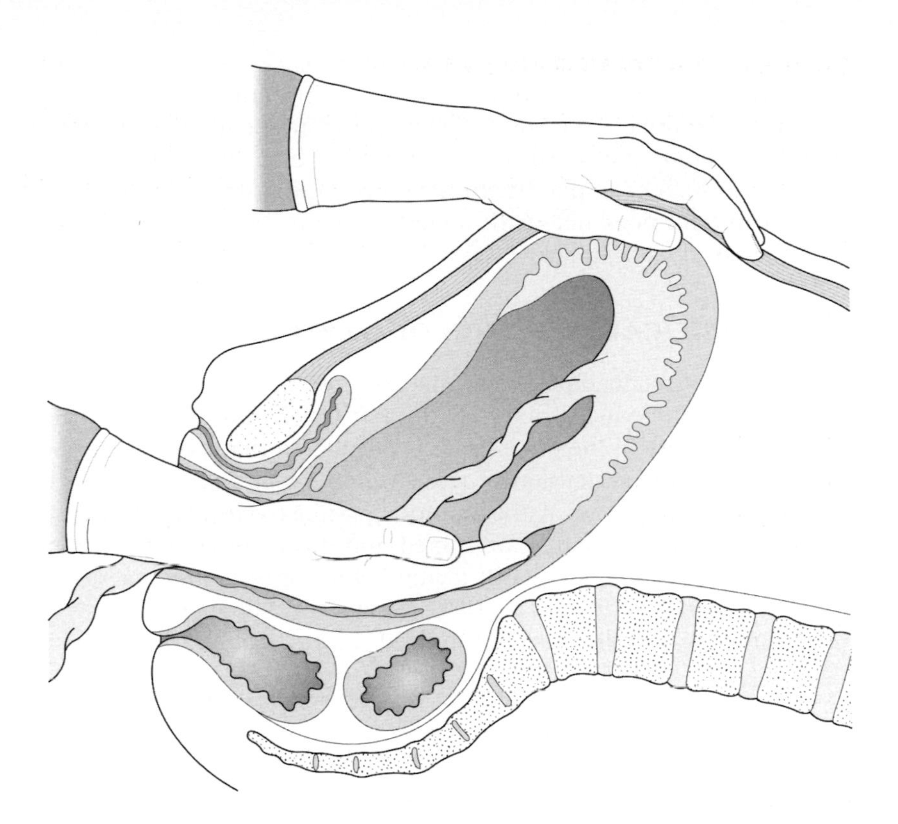

Figure 4.2 Manual removal of the placenta

adherent. Once the placenta has been removed the uterus is re-explored to make sure that there are no remaining placental fragments and that the uterine wall is intact. In those cases where there are small areas of pathological adherence, the placenta should be removed piecemeal from those sites. The cervix and vagina are checked and any lacerations sutured.

An intravenous infusion of oxytocin in crystalloid should be run, to maintain uterine contraction and retraction.

A broad-spectrum antibiotic may be given for 24 hours to prevent infection.

With regional anaesthesia there may not be sufficient uterine relaxation to allow access of the hand into the uterus. In such cases, intravenous glyceryl trinitrate may be used (DeSimone *et al.* 1990; Baskett 1999). See Chapter 9 for details of its administration.

In selected cases when anaesthesia is not in place and the placenta is thought to be retained due to a constriction ring, intravenous glyceryl trinitrate can be used in the hope of allowing spontaneous delivery of the placenta without the need for anaesthesia and manual removal. Obviously, in such cases one has to have everything set up so that if the glyceryl trinitrate does not work anaesthesia can be induced to allow manual removal without delay.

INTRA-UMBILICAL INJECTION OF OXYTOCIN

In some cases of retained placenta, injection into the umbilical cord vein of 10–20 units of oxytocin mixed in 20 ml physiological saline has been used to aid delivery of the placenta. It is postulated that the effect is due to a combination of distension of the chorionic villi and local effect of oxytocin. In the cases studied, the maternal plasma oxytocin levels did not rise. Results of this technique are mixed and inconclusive but it has no adverse effects and may be worth trying before resorting to anaesthesia (Carroli *et al.* 1998; Gazvani *et al.* 1998; Weeks and Mirembe 2002).

The remaining complications of the third stage of labour are covered in Chapter 16.

References

Baskett TF. (1999) Emergency uterine relaxation. In: *Essential Management of Obstetric Emergencies*. 3rd ed. Bristol: Clinical Press. p. 110–14.

Baskett TF. (2000) A flux of the reds: evolution of active management of the third stage of labour. *J R Soc Med* 93:489–93.

Bullough CHW, Msuku RS, Karonde L. (1989) Early suckling and postpartum haemorrhage: controlled trial in deliveries by traditional birth attendants. *Lancet* ii:522–5.

Carroli G, Belizan JM, Grant A, Gonzalez L, Campodonico L, Bergel E. (1998) Intra-umbilical vein injection and retained placenta: evidence from a collaborative large randomised controlled trial. Grupo Argentino de Estudio de Placenta Retenida. *Br J Obstet Gynaecol* 105:178–85.

Choy CMY, Lau WC, Tam WH, Yuen PM. (2002) A randomised controlled trial of intramuscular Syntometrine and intravenous oxytocin in the management of the third stage of labour. *Br J Obstet Gynaecol* 109:173–7.

Chua S, Arulkumaran S, Lim I, Selamat N, Ratnam SS. (1994) Influence of breastfeeding and nipple stimulation on postpartum uterine activity. *Br J Obstet Gynaecol* 101:804–5.

DeSimone CA, Norris MC, Leighton BL. (1990) Intravenous nitroglycerin aids manual extraction of a retained placenta. *Anesthesiology* 73:787–9.

El-Refaey H, O'Brien P, Morafa W, Walder J, Rodeck C. (1997) Use of oral misoprostol in the prevention of postpartum haemorrhage. *Br J Obstet Gynaecol* 104:336–9.

El-Refaey H, Nooh R, O'Brien P. Abdalla M, Geary M, Walder J, Rodeck C. (2000) The misoprostol third stage of labour study: a randomised controlled comparison between orally administered misoprostol and standard management. *Br J Obstet Gynaecol* 107:1104–10.

Gazvani MR, Luckas MJM, Drakeley AJ, Emery SJ, Alfirevic Z, Walkinshaw SA. (1998) Intraumbilical oxytocin for the management of retained placenta: A randomized controlled trial. *Obstet Gynecol* 91:203–7.

Goldberg AB, Greenberg MB, Darney PD. (2001) Misoprostol and pregnancy. *N Engl J Med* 344:38–47.

Granstrom L, Ekman G, Ulmsten U. (1989) Intravenous infusion of 15-methyl prostaglandin F2 alpha (prostinfenem) in women with heavy postpartum hemorrhage. *Acta Obstet Gynecol Scand* 63:365–8.

Gülmezoglu AM, Villar J, Ngoc NT, Piaggio G, Carroli G, Adetoro L, *et al.* (2001) WHO multicentre randomised trial of misoprostol in the management of the third stage of labour. *Lancet* 358:689–95.

Hammar M, Bostrom K, Borgvall B. (1990) Comparison between the influence of methylergometrine and oxytocin on the incidence of retained placenta in the third stage of labour. *Gynecol Obstet Invest* 30:91–4.

Hyashi RH, Castillo LS, Noah ML. (1984) Management of severe postpartum hemorrhage with a prostaglandin F2 alpha analogue. *Obstet Gynecol* 63:806–8.

Kundodyiwa TW, Majoko F, Rusakaniko S. (2001) Misoprostol versus oxytocin in the third stage of labour. *Int J Gynaecol Obstet* 75:235–41.

Ng PS, Chan ASM, Sin WK, Tang LCH, Cheung KB, Yuen PM. (2001) A multicentre randomized controlled trial of oral misoprostol and i.m. Syntometrine in the management of the third stage of labour. *Hum Reprod* 16:31–5.

Nordstrom L, Fogelstam K, Fridman G. (1997) Routine oxytocin in the third stage of labour: placebo controlled randomised trial. *Br J Obstet Gynaecol* 104:781–6.

Oleen MA, Mariano JP. (1990) Controlling refractory atonic postpartum hemorrhage with Hemabate sterile solution. *Am J Obstet Gynecol* 162:205–8.

Paull JD, Ratten GJ. (1977) Ergometrine and third stage blood loss. *Med J Aust* 1:178–9.

Prendiville W, Elbourne D, Chalmers I. (1988) The effect of routine oxytocic administration in the management of the third stage of labour: an overview of the evidence from controlled trials. *Br J Obstet Gynaecol* 95:3–16.

Rogers J, Wood J, McCandlish R, Ayres S, Truesdale A, Elbourne D. (1998) Active versus expectant management of the third stage of labour: the Hinchingbrooke randomised controlled trial. *Lancet* 351:693–9.

Selinger M, MacKenzie I, Dunlop P, James D. (1986) Intra-umbilical vein oxytocin in the management of retained placenta. A double blind controlled study. *J Obstet Gynaecol* 7:115–17.

Soriano D, Dulitzki M, Schiff E, Barkai G, Mashiach S, Seidman DS. (1996) A prospective cohort study of oxytocin plus ergometrine compared with oxytocin alone for prevention of postpartum haemorrhage. *Br J Obstet Gynaecol* 103:1068–73.

Weeks AD, Mirembe FM. (2002) The retained placenta – new insights into an old problem. *Eur J Obstet Gynecol Reprod Biol* 102:109–10.

Yuen PM, Chan NST, Yim SF. (1995) A randomised double-blind comparison of Syntometrine and oxytocin in the management of the third stage of labour. *Br J Obstet Gynaecol* 102:377–80.

5 Induction of labour

Induction of labour is the initiation of uterine contractions to produce effacement and dilatation of the cervix leading to vaginal delivery. In essence, induction of labour is considered when it is felt that the risk(s) to the mother and/or fetus of continuing the pregnancy outweigh the risks of induction and delivery. Induction rates vary greatly between hospitals, depending upon the percentage of high-risk pregnancies, available fetal surveillance and the unit's policies. In the UK, induction rates range from 6–25%, with the average being about 20%.

INDICATIONS FOR INDUCTION OF LABOUR

Potential fetal compromise

The most common indications in this category are prolonged pregnancy (> 41 weeks), hypertensive disorders of pregnancy, intrauterine growth restriction, prelabour rupture of the membranes (PROM) and diabetes.

Maternal indications

Severe pre-eclampsia/eclampsia, antepartum haemorrhage and PROM with chorioamnionitis.

'Soft' indications

There are many 'soft' indications, including: poor obstetric history, psychosocial factors, previous rapid labour and relative geographic isolation. Some of the indications are a combination of both fetal and maternal considerations.

Influencing factors

There are a number of factors in each case that influence the risk of induction and the chance of success. As the indication for many inductions is relative, careful consideration of these influencing factors is necessary.

FACTORS INFLUENCING THE RISK OF INDUCTION

- **Fetal maturity:** Unless the indication is urgent, fetal maturity should be assured before induction is undertaken.
- **Parity:** Multiparous women who have delivered vaginally before are more likely to be successfully induced than the nulliparous woman.
- **State of the cervix:** This is by far the most important consideration in predicting the ease and success of induction. This has been known for centuries but was first quantified by Bishop (1964) in his score, a commonly used modified version of which was proposed by Calder *et al.* (Table 5.1). The station of the fetal head and its application to the cervix are also relevant but the most consistent predictor is the state of the cervix.
- **Additional factors:** Such as previous caesarean section may influence the type of induction (see below).

The most common indication for induction is prolonged pregnancy. Since the post-term trial, induction is offered after 41 completed weeks of gestation, and there is a small but significant reduction of perinatal mortality associated with routine induction after 41 weeks of gestation (Hannah *et al.* 1992; RCOG 2002). However, if the cervix is unfavourable and the woman is fully informed, the alternative of twice weekly fetal surveillance including at least CTG and amniotic fluid assessment may be offered.

As most inductions are not urgent, a careful appraisal of the above factors, which predict the likelihood of success and safety of induction, must be undertaken in each case with the following background question in mind: "Is this induction really necessary?" A properly indicated and conducted induction of labour is justified and safe but it does propel the woman towards a potential cascade of intervention.

Table 5.1 Modified Bishop Score (reproduced with permission from Calder *et al.* 1974)				
Pelvic score	*0*	*1*	*2*	*3*
Position of cervix	Posterior	Middle	Anterior	
Length of cervix (cm)	> 4	3	1–2	< 1
Dilatation of cervix (cm)	0	1–2	3–4	> 4
Consistency of cervix	Firm	Medium	Soft	
Station of presenting part: cm relative to spines	−3	−2	−1/0	+1/+2

Mechanical methods of induction

PRIMING THE CERVIX

The first three techniques described below are generally used to 'prime' or make the cervix more favourable, rather than methods of induction *per se*.

MEMBRANE STRIPPING/SWEEPING

If the cervix is dilated sufficiently to allow one finger to pass, the membranes may be stripped from the internal os and part of the lower uterine segment. This releases endogenous prostaglandins that, over the next few days, will often ripen the cervix. It can, however, be quite uncomfortable for the woman and she should also be warned that it may be followed by a bloodstained discharge. Thus, this is not really a method of inducing labour but it does reduce the numbers of women who have not delivered within one week of membrane stripping (Allott and Palmer 1993). In this context, it may have a role in preventing the need for induction of labour in women who go past their due date. It may also be useful to carry out this procedure when assessing the cervix a day or two before planned induction. Although it is uncomfortable for the woman, it has not been shown to have any deleterious maternal or neonatal effects.

HYGROSCOPIC DILATORS

These are placed in the cervix and absorb water, thus causing mechanical dilatation. The naturally occurring *Laminaria japonica* may cause infection, so a synthetic polyvinyl sponge impregnated with magnesium sulphate (Lamicel®, MedGyn) is preferable. These are introduced through the internal os 12 hours before induction. They may improve the Bishop score but there is no proof that they enhance the outcome of induction.

CATHETERS

The most commonly used is the Foley catheter, which has been shown to improve the Bishop score. The catheter is placed through the internal os and the balloon inflated with 30 ml of saline. A catheter may be used as an alternative to prostaglandins when these are contraindicated, such as in patients with asthma. In addition, it is much cheaper than the prostaglandin gels.

AMNIOTOMY

In the presence of a favourable cervix, amniotomy is the most effective method of induction and approximately 80–90% of women will come into labour within 24 hours after amniotomy alone. Its efficacy and the induction to delivery interval are greatly improved by starting intravenous oxytocin at or soon after the amniotomy.

Medical methods of induction

OXYTOCIN

In the presence of an unfavourable cervix and with intact membranes, oxytocin is ineffective. However, once the membranes are ruptured, and particularly if the cervix is favourable, oxytocin is a very effective adjunct to induction of labour. Oxytocin can be diluted in either crystalloid or 5% dextrose-saline. The starting dose is 1–2 milliunits/minute and the dosage increased until effective contractions are established. Studies of the half-life of oxytocin and dose increment interval suggest that a 30-minute interval between increasing doses is the most effective while reducing the risk of hyperstimulation. Uterine contractions and fetal heart rate should be monitored during induction of labour. However, it is not necessary to use sophisticated automatic infusion systems or intrauterine pressure monitoring (Chia *et al.* 1993). A suggested dosage schedule from the National Institute of Clinical Excellence is shown in Table 5.2.

PROSTAGLANDINS

Prostaglandins have been used by the oral, intravenous, intracervical and vaginal routes with varying degrees of success. Because of adverse effects, or lack of efficacy compared with oxytocin, the oral and intravenous routes have largely been discontinued apart from in trials with the use of the oral prostaglandin E_1 analogue misoprostol (see below).

Table 5. 2 Oxytocin infusion protocol for induction of labour (NICE 2001)			
Time (minutes)	*Oxytocin dose (milliunits/ minute)*	*Dilution 30 iu oxytocin in 500 ml normal saline ml/hour*	*Dilution 10 iu in oxytocin 500 ml normal saline ml/hour*
0	1	1	3
30	2	2	6
60	4	4	12
90	8	8	24
120	12	12	36
150	16	16	48
180	20	20	60
210	24	24	72
240	28	28	84
270	32	32	96

Prostaglandin E_2 (dinoprostone)

Dinoprostone has been used in a dose of 0.5 mg intracervically but this has no advantages over the vaginal route and is a little more difficult to administer (Hales *et al.* 1994). The dose of prostaglandin E_2 vaginal gel or tablets is 1 mg or 2 mg (Nuutila and Kajanoja 1996; Rix *et al.* 1996). Usually the 2-mg dose is given to the nulliparous woman and the 1-mg dose to the multiparous woman. Dosage intervals may be 6–12 hours and up to three applications can be given. The other prostaglandin E_2 is a 10-mg dose in a vaginal insert with slow release at a rate of 0.3 mg per hour (Smith *et al.* 1994). This insert also has a tape attached to it so that it can be removed in the case of hyperstimulation.

Prostaglandin E_1 analogue (misoprostol)

This prostaglandin is under investigation and shows promise both by the oral and vaginal routes (Shetty *et al.* 2001; Sanchez-Ramos *et al.* 2002). The vaginal route seems to be more effective and the dose varies from 25–50 μg. There may be a slightly increased risk of uterine hyperstimulation. It is at least as effective, and in some cases more so, than vaginal prostaglandin E_2 gel.

In terms of cost, oxytocin and misoprostol are cheap, whereas the other prostaglandins are much more expensive. The main role for the prostaglandins is with the unfavourable cervix. The most commonly used agent is vaginal prostaglandin E_2 but this may be superseded by the much less expensive misoprostol when clinical trials have defined the most appropriate and safest route and dose. For the favourable cervix, amniotomy and oxytocin is the most cost-effective method. It is important that individual units establish their own selection criteria for induction of labour and develop management protocols for patients with the favourable and unfavourable cervix.

Special circumstances

PREVIOUS CAESAREAN SECTION

In patients with a previous single, low-transverse caesarean section, induction of labour may be undertaken with amniotomy and oxytocin. If the cervix is unfavourable and prostaglandins have to be considered, induction should only be carried out for strong indications as this will increase the risk of uterine rupture (Ravisa *et al.* 2000; Lydon-Rochelle *et al.* 2001). The woman must be told of this increased risk. Such cases should prompt a careful appraisal and answers to the two questions:

- Is this induction really necessary?
- Why am I not doing a repeat elective caesarean section?

Misoprostol has been shown to increase the risk of uterine rupture after previous caesarean section to a high degree in small series and should not be used for this purpose (Plaut *et al.* 1998; Wing *et al.* 1998).

INTRAUTERINE FETAL DEATH

In the vast majority of these tragic cases the woman wishes to have labour induced and this request should be honoured if possible. The guiding principle is to make the induction and subsequent labour as smooth and humane as possible. Ironically, this is to some extent made easier by the fact that potential fetal adverse effects of the induction agents are not a consideration. Unless the cervix is very favourable, so that amniotomy and oxytocin are likely to succeed, prostaglandins are the best choice (Kent *et al.* 1984). In this context, misoprostol has much to offer as it can be given both orally and vaginally (Bugalho *et al.* 1994). An essential aspect of these cases is the time taken with the woman and her partner to emphasise that some time may be required for the prostaglandins to ripen the cervix and initiate labour. Without this explanation and support, one or both partners may become so distraught that they seek elective caesarean section as refuge from their anguish – thus increasing the risk to the woman now and in any future pregnancy.

STABILISING INDUCTION

In some women with a transverse or oblique lie there is an indication for induction of labour. In such cases, external cephalic version is performed and the head guided over the pelvic brim. An intravenous infusion of oxytocin is started and, when contractions are established and strong enough, amniotomy is performed. It is important to hold the head over the brim and release a fair amount of amniotic fluid so that the head is well stabilised on the lower segment and cervix and will be held there by the uterine activity. A variation of this principle may also be performed when the head is free and mobile at the pelvic brim. This approach reduces the chance of cord prolapse.

Complications of induction of labour

FAILED INDUCTION

If the indication for induction of labour is urgent then failed induction will have to be resolved by caesarean section. This is perfectly acceptable when the indication for induction is strong. In many cases, however, the indication for induction is 'soft' and, after attempted ripening of the cervix with prostaglandins, there is no progress but both the mother and fetus are well. In such cases, a careful review of the situation with the parents may allow one to 'back off' and, with fetal surveillance, try a repeat induction hours or even days later. Such cases should always harden one's resolve to be careful in the selection of patients for induction of labour.

FETAL IMMATURITY

Provided accurate ultrasound has been carried out in the first half of pregnancy this should not occur. In the small number of cases when delivery of the fetus is necessary regardless of maturity, this will have to be accepted. In borderline cases, amniocentesis to assess fetal lung maturity and/or administration of antenatal corticosteroids may be necessary.

UTERINE HYPERSTIMULATION

This can potentially lead to fetal hypoxia and even death. Before induction it is wise to obtain a fetal heart rate tracing and only if this is normal, proceed with oxytocic stimulation. In the case of prostaglandins, the fetal heart rate should be monitored during uterine activity. If there is hyperstimulation, the prostaglandin gel or tablet should be washed out of the vagina and, if necessary, tocolysis in the form of subcutaneous terbutaline 0.25 mg administered together with the usual first-aid management of turning the woman on to her side and administering oxygen. The half-life of oxytocin is so short that hyperstimulation in response to this agent is usually quickly corrected by discontinuing the infusion.

CORD PROLAPSE

This is a potential risk, particularly if the presenting part is poorly applied to the lower uterine segment and cervix. The precautions mentioned above with stabilising induction are relevant. In general, however, this risk is overstated and, provided that reasonable care is taken during amniotomy, the risk of cord prolapse need not be increased (Roberts *et al.* 1997).

PLACENTAL ABRUPTION

Amniotomy in cases of polyhydramnios may lead to such rapid decompression of the uterus that placental abruption may occur. This is quite rare provided the amniotic fluid is slowly released by controlling the head with one hand. In cases where there is marked polyhydramnios it may be prudent to perform amniocentesis and withdraw fluid abdominally until the polyhydramnios is relieved and the presenting part well stabilised over the pelvic brim.

CHORIOAMNIONITIS

Once amniotomy is performed this risk increases. This can be kept to a minimum by starting intravenous oxytocin at or shortly after the time of amniotomy to reduce the induction to delivery interval.

ELECTROLYTE IMBALANCE

Prolonged high doses of oxytocin in dilute solutions can lead to maternal water intoxication and hyponatraemia. If the recommended infusion schedules are followed, this should not occur.

POSTPARTUM HAEMORRHAGE

There is an increased risk of uterine atony following oxytocic induction of labour. This can be prevented by active management of the third stage of labour and the provision of an oxytocic agent for six to eight hours postpartum.

NEONATAL HYPERBILIRUBINAEMIA

The use of oxytocin for induction of labour has been associated with an increased incidence of neonatal jaundice in some studies, but this does not constitute a clinical threat to the neonate.

Conclusion

Induction of labour is one of the most common and beneficial obstetric interventions, provided that it is undertaken for valid indications and with careful selection and application of the appropriate method (ACOG 1999; SOGC 2001; RCOG 2002). It is, however, not without risk and it is still probably wise to reflect on the words of Sir Alexander Turnbull 25 years ago: "The spontaneous onset of labour is a robust and effective mechanism ... We should only induce labour when we are sure that we can do better".

References

Allott HA, Palmer CR. (1993) Sweeping the membranes: a valid procedure in stimulating the onset of labour? *Br J Obstet Gynaecol* 100:898–903.

American College of Obstetricians and Gynecologists (1999). *Practice Bulletin No. 10: Induction of Labor*. Washington DC: ACOG.

Bishop EH. (1964) Pelvic scoring for elective induction. *Obstet Gynecol* 2:266–8.

Bugalho A, Bique C, Machungo F, Faaundes A. (1994) Induction of labor with intravaginal misoprostol and intrauterine fetal death. *Am J Obstet Gynecol* 171:538–41.

Calder AA, Embrey MP, Hillier K. (1974) Extra-amniotic prostaglandin E2 for the induction of labour. *J Obstet Gynaecol Br Cwlth* 81:39–46.

Chia YT, Arulkumaran S, Soon SB, Norshida S, Ratnam SS. (1993) Induction of labour: Does internal tocography result in better obstetric outcome than external tocography? *Aust N Z J Obstet Gynaecol* 33:159–61.

Hales KA, Rayburn WF, Turnbull GL, Christensen HD, Patatanian E. (1994) Double-blind comparison of intracervical and intravaginal prostaglandin E2 for cervical ripening and induction of labor. *Am J Obstet Gynecol* 171:1087–91.

Hannah ME, Hannah WJ, Hellman J, Hewson S, Milner R, William A. (1992) Induction of labor as compared with serial antenatal monitoring in post-term pregnancy. A randomised controlled trial. *N Engl J Med* 326:1587–92.

Kent DR, Goldstein AI, Linzey EM. (1984) Safety and efficacy of vaginal prostaglandin E2 suppositories in the management of the third-trimester fetal demise. *J Reprod Med* 29:101–2.

Lydon-Rochelle M, Holt VL, Easterling TR, Martin DP. (2001) Risk of uterine rupture during labor among women with a prior cesarean delivery. *N Engl J Med* 345:3–8.

National Institute of Clinical Excellence (NICE). (2001) *Induction of labour. Clinical Guideline D*. London: NICE.

Nuutila M, Kajanoja P. (1996) Local administration of prostaglandin E1 for cervical ripening and labor induction: the appropriate route and dose. *Acta Obstet Gynecol Scand* 75:135–8.

Plaut MN, Schwartz ML, Lubarsky SL. (1998) Uterine rupture associated with the use of misoprostol in the gravid patient with a previous cesarean section. *Am J Obstet Gynecol* 180:1535–42.

Ravisa DJ, Wood SL, Pollard JK. (2000) Uterine rupture during induced trial of labor among women with previous cesarean delivery. *Am J Obstet Gynecol* 183:1176–9.

Rix P, Ladehoff P, Motler AM, Tilma KA, Zdravkovic M. (1996) Cervical ripening and induction of delivery by local administration of prostaglandin E2 gel or vaginal tablets is equally effective. *Acta Obstet Gynecol Scand* 75:45–7.

Roberts WA, Martin RW, Roach HH, Perry KG, Martin JN, Morrison JC. (1997) Are obstetric interventions such as cervical ripening, induction of labor, amnioinfusion, or amniotomy associated with umbilical cord prolapse? *Am J Obstet Gynecol* 176:1181–5.

Royal College of Obstetricians and Gynaecologists (RCOG). (2002) *Induction of Labour. Evidence-based Clinical Guideline No. 9*. London: RCOG Press.

Sanchez-Ramos L, Kaunitz AM, Delka I. (2002) Labor induction with 25 mg versus 50 mg intravaginal misoprostol: a systematic review. *Obstet Gynecol* 99:145–51.

Shetty A, Danielian P, Templeton A. (2001) A comparison of oral and vaginal misoprostol tablets in induction of labour at term. *Br J Obstet Gynaecol* 108:238–43.

Smith CV, Rayburn WF, Miller AM. (1994) Intravaginal prostaglandin E2 for cervical ripening and initiation of labor. Comparison of a multidose gel and single, controlled-release pessary. *J Reprod Med* 39:381–4.

Wing DA, Lovett K, Paul RH. (1998) Disruption of prior uterine incision following misoprostol labor induction in women with previous cesarean delivery. *Obstet Gynecol* 91:828–30.

Society of Obstetricians and Gynaecologists of Canada. (2001) Induction of Labour at Term. Clinical Practice Guidelines No. 107. *J Obstet Gynaecol Can* 23:717–28.

6 Preterm labour and prelabour rupture of membranes

Preterm birth with its associated complications contributes disproportionately to perinatal mortality and morbidity. Defined as delivery before 37 completed weeks, preterm labour occurs in 6–9% of all deliveries. In developed countries, preterm births lead to about 70% of neonatal deaths and 50% of childhood neurological disabilities. The incidence of severe handicap in those born before 28 weeks of gestation is about 10%, with a greater percentage having moderate to minor disabilities (Wood *et al.* 2000). About two-thirds of preterm deliveries occur between 34 and 37 weeks of gestation and, with modern perinatal care, this group usually has a good outcome. The main morbidity and mortality is within the group that deliver below 34 weeks. At 34–37 weeks, many cases of preterm birth are iatrogenic, having been induced or delivered by elective caesarean section for maternal and/or fetal indications. Below 34 weeks of gestation only a small number of cases are iatrogenic.

Aetiology

The cause of spontaneous preterm labour is often not apparent and may be multifactorial. There are a number of associations:

- demographic and socio-economic factors
- reproductive history
- uterine factors
- infection.

The prediction of preterm labour is imperfect, as the majority of cases do not have any of the above risk factors. The main associations are in the past history of preterm labour, second-trimester delivery (spontaneous or induced) and multiple pregnancy (ACOG 2001).

DEMOGRAPHIC AND SOCIO-ECONOMIC FACTORS

The main correlations are with the following factors:

- extremes of maternal age (less than 17 years and over 35 years)
- low socio-economic class
- unmarried
- low prepregnancy weight
- smoking (Kolas *et al.* 2000)
- cocaine use
- anaemia.

However, the relationship between these factors and spontaneous preterm labour is neither sensitive nor specific enough to be of great clinical value.

REPRODUCTIVE HISTORY

Those with a previous history of spontaneous preterm labour or second-trimester miscarriage, particularly more than one episode, have an increased risk of subsequent preterm labour. Induced abortion in the first trimester is not a major factor but later second-trimester induced abortions may increase the risk (Henriet and Kaminski 2001). Overall, about 10% of cases of spontaneous preterm labour have such a past history.

UTERINE FACTORS

- Congenital uterine anomalies and uterine fibroids only slightly increase the risk of preterm labour.
- Cervical weakness, either idiopathic or secondary to surgical trauma or *in utero* exposure to diethylstilboestrol, is a rare contributor to preterm delivery.
- Uterine overdistension associated with multiple pregnancy and/or polyhydramnios increases the risk of preterm delivery.

INFECTION

There is an inconsistent link between maternal cervical and vaginal infections and spontaneous preterm labour and prelabour rupture of the membranes. These may include ureaplasma, *Trichomonas vaginalis* and bacterial vaginosis. A number of these infections are linked with socio-economic factors, so the correlation is unclear. There is a small association with urinary tract infection, particularly pyelonephritis, and preterm labour.

Diagnosis

CLINICAL

The diagnosis may be obvious, with regular, painful contractions associated with progressive cervical effacement and dilatation. On other occasions the symptoms may be non-specific, such as uterine cramping, backache and increased vaginal discharge. There may or may not be a show or rupture of membranes. Digital examination of cervical effacement and dilatation is subjective and can differ between examiners.

The clinical dilemma is that by the time the symptoms and signs of labour are obvious treatment will probably not be effective. Thus, over-diagnosis and treatment of preterm labour is understandably common.

ULTRASOUND

Transvaginal cervical sonography can be a useful predictor of the likelihood of preterm labour and has been shown to be superior to digital examination alone (Gomez *et al.* 1994). The vaginal probe assesses the length of the cervix as well as the presence or absence of funnelling.

FIBRONECTIN

Fetal fibronectin is the extracellular matrix protein that causes adherence of the fetal membranes to the adjacent uterine decidua. High levels of fibronectin in the cervicovaginal secretions may indicate disruption of that membrane–decidual bond and represent an increased risk of preterm labour and delivery. Review of the clinical trials using this test shows that its main benefit may be its very high negative predictive value (Shellhaas and Iames 2001).

Management

Depending upon the facilities available, the following initial appraisal is carried out:

- history and physical examination to establish the gestational age, estimated fetal weight, lie and presentation
- a pelvic examination, including speculum, to assess the length and dilatation of the cervix, take appropriate swabs for culture (e.g. group B streptococcus) and the fetal fibronectin test (if available)
- transvaginal ultrasound to assess the length, dilatation and funnelling of the cervix
- transabdominal ultrasound to assess the number of fetuses,

presentation, lie, amount of amniotic fluid and anatomical normality of the fetus
- cardiotocography
- midstream urine culture.

If the woman is at or over 34 weeks of gestation, no attempts to stop labour or administer corticosteroids and tocolytics need be undertaken. Similarly, at an earlier gestation, if conditions necessitate delivery of the fetus (e.g. placental abruption) then labour and delivery should be allowed to continue.

CORTICOSTEROIDS

There is now widespread experience with the use of corticosteroids to reduce neonatal hyaline membrane disease and respiratory distress (NIH Consensus Development Panel 1995). These may be given up to 34 weeks of gestation and are especially beneficial before 32 weeks. The dose is betamethasone 12 mg intramuscularly, 12 hours apart. For full benefit, 48 hours should pass after administration of the last dose. However, there is some benefit even 24 hours after administration. In women who do not proceed to delivery, there is controversy as to whether repeated corticosteroid doses should be given at regular intervals. Until the safety and benefit of repeated doses is established this practice should be confined to clinical trials (NIH Consensus Development Panel 2001; ACOG 2002).

ANTIBIOTICS

The routine use of antibiotics in women with threatened preterm labour has not been shown to prolong gestation or improve perinatal outcome (Kenyon *et al.* 2001a).

However, for those women who do proceed in preterm labour to delivery the risk of neonatal group B streptococcus is increased. Thus, once labour is definitely established, many will treat prophylactically with penicillin G or, if allergic, erythromycin.

TOCOLYTICS

In cases below 32 weeks of gestation and in selected women of 32–34 weeks, tocolytic treatment is given. The main benefit of tocolysis, which has only been shown to be effective for up to 48 hours, is to use that time to administer and allow corticosteroids to take effect and/or transfer the woman to a tertiary care centre if needed.

There are a number of tocolytics in use or under investigation. All of these agents have contraindications and potentially serious adverse effects. Each unit should establish their own detailed protocol. The administration of the more common of these agents is outlined on page 58.

Labour and delivery

If preterm labour occurs after 34 weeks, if tocolysis fails, or after 48 hours administration of tocolysis and corticosteroids, labour is allowed to continue.

If the fetus is in cephalic presentation, labour is allowed to continue and managed as in term labour. Continuous electronic fetal heart rate monitoring is advisable as the premature infant is more vulnerable to hypoxia. The vacuum extractor should not be used on the premature fetal head and prophylactic forceps are not required. A gently controlled delivery of the fetal head is necessary and episiotomy may be performed if there is soft-tissue resistance from the perineum.

If the fetus is in breech presentation, although there is no clear evidence to support it, most obstetricians will proceed to delivery by caesarean section. Depending upon the development of the lower uterine segment, a low transverse incision may be made but tocolysis with glyceryl trinitrate or terbutaline should be drawn up and ready to administer to assist delivery of the aftercoming head, which is proportionately much larger than the body in the premature fetus (see Chapter 9).

The medical, ethical and financial aspects of perinatal intervention and intensive care of the preterm infant are considerable (McClure and Bell 2001). Unfortunately, modern neonatal intensive care produces both more intact and more handicapped survivors. Thus, the gestation at which one intervenes between 25 and 27 weeks must be carefully considered in the context of the available neonatal facilities and the understanding and wishes of the couple.

Prelabour rupture of membranes

The spontaneous rupture of membranes during labour is normal. In about 10% of term pregnancies the membranes rupture spontaneously before the onset of labour (term PROM). In about 30–40% of cases of preterm labour (less than 37 weeks) the membranes rupture before the onset of labour (preterm PROM).

AETIOLOGY

In most cases there is no obvious cause.

TOCOLYTIC AGENTS

- **Beta-adrenergic agonists (ritodrine, terbutaline, salbutamol)**
  These agents act on the beta-adrenoreceptors and the following potential serious adverse effects can occur: cardiac arrhythmia, tachycardia and ischaemia; hypotension; pulmonary oedema; glycogenolysis leading to hyperglycaemia (contraindicated in diabetes); hypokalaemia.
  Ritodrine is given by intravenous infusion starting with 100 μg/minute and increasing by 50 μg/minute every 15 minutes until the contractions cease or up to a maximum rate of 350 μg/minute, provided that adverse effects do not occur. The dose should be reduced or stopped if the maternal pulse rate is greater than 120 bpm.
  Terbutaline is given subcutaneously in the dose of 0.15–0.5 mg every four hours.
- **Prostaglandin synthetase inhibitors (indomethacin)**
  These drugs inhibit the cyclo-oxygenase (COX) enzymes COX-1 and COX-2 that are important in the synthesis of prostaglandins. The dose of indomethacin is 25–50 mg orally or rectally every six hours. Unfortunately, indomethacin, while an effective tocolytic, has been shown to have significant fetal adverse effects including: intracranial haemorrhage, closure of patent ductus arteriosus and necrotising enterocolitis (Macones *et al.* 2001). In future selective COX-2 inhibitors may be effective with fewer adverse effects and the results of clinical trials are awaited.
- **Calcium channel blockers (nifedipine)**
  These appears to be as or more effective than beta-adrenergic agonists and with fewer adverse effects. Nifedipine inhibits the influx of calcium ions through cell membrane via calcium channels. It may cause transient maternal hypotension. The dose is 10–20 mg orally every four to six hours (Tsatsaris *et al.* 2001).
- **Oxytocin antagonists (atosiban)**
  These drugs may have similar efficacy to the beta-adrenergic agonists but with fewer adverse effects. Atosiban is given as an initial 6.75 mg intravenously, followed by 300 μg/minute intravenously for three hours and maintained at 100 μg/minute for 48 hours (Worldwide Atosiban Study Group 2001).
- **Glycerol trinitrate**
  This nitric oxide donor is under study, using 10 mg slow-release skin patches.

- The role of bacterial colonisation and infection of the vagina and cervix in PROM is suspected but unclear. Infections such as bacterial vaginosis, mycoplasma and ureaplasma may alter the vaginal pH or produce proteases that weaken the membranes.
- Increased intra-amniotic pressure associated with multiple pregnancy or polyhydramnios may be implicated.
- Potentially traumatic procedures such as amniocentesis and external cephalic version are rare causes.
- An incompetent cervix may expose the membranes to the vaginal flora and this, together with lack of support at the internal os, may lead to rupture of the membranes. Overall, this is a rare cause.

DIAGNOSIS

The history is often clear, with the sudden uncontrolled loss of clear fluid from the vagina. Others may have a less dramatic clear discharge.

On sterile speculum examination the diagnosis may be obvious, with fluid draining through the cervix and pooling in the posterior fornix.

A piece of nitrazine paper placed in the fluid will turn blue if it is alkaline, suggesting that it is amniotic fluid. Normal urine and vaginal secretions are acidic and the paper will not turn blue. However, false positives can be obtained with antiseptics, blood, serum and semen.

The definitive test, if positive, is ferning. A drop of the fluid is placed on a clean slide, allowed to dry, examined under the microscope and, if positive, ferning due to crystals of sodium and potassium chloride will be seen. Ferning can be inhibited by blood and serum so that false negatives can occur. However, if ferning is seen then the presence of amniotic fluid is confirmed.

Abdominal examination should include the estimated fetal weight, presentation and lie. Uterine irritability and tenderness may presage chorioamnionitis.

Ultrasound assessment should include an anatomical survey for fetal anomaly, if this has not already been done, and to rule out cord presentation/prolapse. An assessment of the amniotic fluid volume will be helpful, especially if conservative management is undertaken. In cases where the history and speculum examination leave doubt about the diagnosis the finding of a normal amount of amniotic fluid and, particularly fluid below the presenting part, may help rule out ruptured membranes.

In selected cases, fluid may be taken from the posterior fornix and sent for laboratory assessment of fetal lung maturity. Cervical and vaginal swabs can be taken for culture. No digital examination should be performed as this may increase the risk of infection.

Prelabour rupture of membranes at term

In 80% of women with term PROM, labour is established within 24 hours and in 90% within 48 hours.

In general, induction of labour is indicated with term PROM. However, the timing may be delayed if the woman wishes. Depending on the availability of facilities there is much to be said for waiting 12 hours as half the women will be in spontaneous labour by that time. Most women prefer to wait only 24 hours before induction if spontaneous labour does not occur. Intravenous oxytocin as the method of induction is preferred over prostaglandins (Enkin *et al.* 2000), although oral misoprostol may have a role when clinical trials are complete (Ngai *et al.* 2000).

If there are signs of chorioamnionitis at the time of diagnosis, labour should be induced and covered with a broad-spectrum antibiotic such as ampicillin. If the woman is group B streptococcus positive, or if the membranes are ruptured more than 24 hours, penicillin prophylaxis should be given (Hannah *et al.* 1997).

Preterm prelabour rupture of membranes

In preterm PROM, the aim is to gain time for fetal maturity. Between 35 and 37 weeks of gestation, consideration may be given to induction of labour.

MANAGEMENT

The patient is observed in hospital for clinical signs of infection including pyrexia, uterine tenderness and irritability, together with a purulent vaginal discharge. Unfortunately, early warning laboratory tests such as, daily white-cell counts and C-reactive protein have not been found to have practical clinical application. If chorioamnionitis develops, start intravenous antibiotics and deliver the patient either by induction of labour or caesarean section depending on the clinical findings. In many women, one of the earliest signs of chorioamnionitis is the onset of labour.

Antibiotics have been shown to prolong the pregnancy, reduce maternal infection and decrease neonatal morbidity (Kenyon *et al.* 2001b). The most common regimen is a seven-day course of erythromycin or amoxicillin.

If the gestation is between 24 and 32 weeks, corticosteroids should be given as for preterm labour.

In general, tocolytic treatment is not indicated or effective in preterm PROM. However, in the face of threatened preterm labour without signs of chorioamnionitis it may be used for up to 48 hours to allow corticosteroids to take effect and/or transfer the woman to a tertiary care unit. In most cases of preterm PROM, when labour threatens tocolysis is unsuccessful.

In many cases, labour does not supervene and a number of weeks are gained. During this time, the fetus should be assessed by ultrasound for growth every two weeks. Amniotic fluid volume assessment should be carried out twice a week. There is a risk of pulmonary hypoplasia and positional limb deformities in the fetus should chronic oligohydramnios persist. There is a small but increased risk of placental abruption in preterm PROM. Cardiotocography and biophysical profile may be carried out weekly or more often when a gestation is reached at which one is willing to act upon the results.

If the pregnancy is safely carried to 35–37 weeks of gestation, depending on the presence or absence of oligohydramnios and other aspects of fetal growth and oxygenation, induction of labour may be discussed with the parents.

References

ACOG. (2001) *Practice Bulletin No. 31. Assessment of Risk Factors for Preterm Birth.* Washington DC: American College of Obstetricians and Gynecologists.

ACOG. (2002) *Committee Opinion No. 273. Antenatal Corticosteroid Therapy for Fetal Maturation.* Washington DC: American College of Obstetricians and Gynecologists.

Enkin M, Keirse MJNC, Neilson J, Crowther C, Duley L, Hodnett E, Hofmeyr J. (2000) Prelabor rupture of membranes. In: *A Guide to Effective Care in Pregnancy and Childbirth.* 3rd ed. Oxford: Oxford University Press. p. 196–210.

Gomez R, Glasso M, Romero R. (1994) Ultrasonographic examination of the uterus cervix is better than cervical digital examination as a predictor of the likelihood of premature delivery in patients with preterm labour and intact membranes. *Am J Obstet Gynecol* 171:956–4.

Hannah ME, Ohlsson A, Wang EE, Matlow A, Foster GA, Willan AR, *et al.* (1997) Maternal colonization with group B streptococcus and prelabour rupture of membranes at term: the role of induction of labour. Term PROM Study group. *Am J Obstet Gynecol* 177:780–5.

Henriet L, Kaminski M. (2001) Impact of induced abortions on subsequent pregnancy outcome: the 1995 French national perinatal survey. *Br J Obstet Gynaecol* 108:1036–42.

Kenyon SL, Taylor DJ, Tarnow-Mordi W. (2001a) Broad spectrum antibiotics for spontaneous preterm labour: the ORACLE II randomized trial. ORACLE Collaborative Group. *Lancet* 357:989–94.

Kenyon SL, Taylor DJ, Tarnow-Mordi W. (2001b) Broad-spectrum antibiotics for preterm, prelabour rupture of fetal membranes: the ORACLE I randomized trial. ORACLE Collaborative Group. *Lancet* 357:979–88.

Kolas T, Nakling J, Salvesen KA. (2000) Smoking during pregnancy increases the risks of preterm births among parous women. *Acta Obstet Gynecol Scand* 79:644–8.

McClure BG, Bell AH. (2001) The edge of viability. In: Sturdee D, Oláh K, Keane D, editors. *Yearbook of Obstetrics and Gynaecology Volume 9*. London: RCOG Press. p.288–94.

Macones GA, Marder SJ, Clothier B, Stamilio DM. (2001) The controversy surrounding indomethacin for tocolysis. *Am J Obstet Gynecol* 184:264–72.

Ngai N, Chen Y, Lam S. (2000) Misoprostol vs oxytocin in prelabor rupture of membranes. *Br J Obstet Gynaecol* 107:222–7.

NIH Consensus Development Panel. (1995) Effect of corticosteroids for fetal maturation on perinatal outcomes. *JAMA* 273:413–8.

NIH Consensus Development Panel. (2001) Antenatal corticosteroids revisited. *Obstet Gynecol* 98:144–50.

Shellhaas CS, Iames JD. (2001) The diagnosis and management of preterm labour. *J Obstet Gynaecol Res* 27:305–11.

Tsatsaris V, Papatsonis D, Goffinet F, Dekker G, Carbonne B. (2001) Tocolysis with nifedipine or beta-adrenergic agonists: a meta-analysis. *Obstet Gynecol* 97:840–47.

Wood NS, Marlow N, Costeloe K, Gibson AT, Wilkinson AR. EPICure Study Group. (2000) Neurologic and developmental disability after extremely preterm birth. *N Engl J Med* 343:378–84.

Worldwide Atosiban versus Beta-agonists Study Group. Effectiveness and safety of the oxytocin antagonist atosiban versus beta-adrenergic agonists in the treatment of preterm labour. *Br J Obstet Gynaecol* 108:133–42.

7 Assisted vaginal delivery

Rates of assisted vaginal delivery with forceps and vacuum vary from country to country and within countries from hospital to hospital. The range may be from 4% to 26% but is commonly between 5% and 15% of all deliveries (Drife 1996). Similarly, the use of forceps and vacuum varies greatly between and within countries. Some units will use one or other instrument almost exclusively but, overall, the use of the vacuum is increasing (Hillier and Johanson 1994; Bofill *et al.* 1996; Hankins and Rowe 1996).

DEFINITION OF ASSISTED PELVIC DELIVERY

The American College of Obstetricians and Gynecologists provides the following working definitions:

- **Outlet delivery** The fetal head is at or on the perineum and the scalp is visible without separating the labia. The head is either direct OA or OP or less than 45° off the anteroposterior diameter.
- **Low pelvis** The outlet criteria are not fulfilled but the head is at least at station +2 cm. Thc position may bc OA, OT or OP.
- **Mid pelvis** The fetal head is at the level of the ischial spines to spines +1 cm.

Indications

There are few absolute indications for assisted vaginal delivery: most indications are relative and fall into the following broad categories:

- maternal
- fetal
- combined.

MATERNAL

- Fatigue and exhaustion may lead to unproductive and non-progressive maternal effort.
- A medical condition may limit the desirability of maternal effort, e.g. cardiac, cerebrovascular disease, severe pre-eclampsia.
- Maternal request.

FETAL

- Fetal distress, manifest by abnormal fetal heart rate or cord prolapse. In these circumstances it is essential that the assisted vaginal delivery be straightforward, as the combination of trauma and hypoxia is potentially damaging to the fetus.

COMBINED

In a prolonged, non-progressive second stage of labour the indication to intervene is based on a balance of maternal and fetal reasons. Often the mother is exhausted, possibly demoralised, and her efforts are non-progressive. Prolongation may cause damage to the maternal pelvic floor. The position of the fetal head: deflexed occipitotransverse or occipitoposterior, may present a larger diameter, contributing to the relative disproportion. Assisted vaginal delivery that corrects this deflexion will lead to a smaller diameter and easy delivery. Prolonged arrest of the fetal head may lead to the lethal combination of fetal trauma and hypoxia. It has been suggested that, when the following times are exceeded in the second stage of labour, consideration should be given to assisted delivery (ACOG 2000).

- nullipara – two hours without regional anaesthesia and three hours with regional anaesthesia
- multipara – one hour without regional anaesthesia and two hours with regional anaesthesia.

However, no rigid time limits should be applied, as a combination of some or all of the above maternal and fetal factors, together with balanced judgement, is needed to define the correct time for intervention.

Conditions to be fulfilled for assisted vaginal delivery

INDICATION AND CONSENT

In the often highly charged environment of the labour ward it can be difficult to obtain informed consent. However, the broad options, which usually include waiting, assisted vaginal delivery or caesarean section, should be discussed with the patient. It is important to document this and the indication for intervention (RCOG 2000).

EFFECTIVE POWERS

One of the most important principles put forward by O'Driscoll *et al.* (1993) is that propulsion is more effective and safer than traction and extraction. Thus, it is essential to use the uterine and maternal powers to best effect before resorting to assisted delivery. The principles of appropriate oxytocin augmentation and use of maternal effort are outlined in Chapter 2.

COMBINED ABDOMINAL/VAGINAL ASSESSMENT

A most important principle is that neither abdominal nor vaginal assessment alone provides adequate information upon which to base the decision to assist vaginal delivery (Knight *et al.* 1993). In particular, the relationship of the leading bony part of the fetal head to the ischial spines (station) can be misleading with vaginal examination alone because of the difficulties in assessing the contribution of caput and moulding to the true level of descent (Figure 7.1). In this context, the principle of assessing the fetal head in 'fifths' above the pelvic brim is important, as outlined in Chapter 2. In general, if the fetal head is not palpable above the pelvic brim, the head has descended to at least spines +1 to +2 cm. In modern obstetrics it is rarely indicated to assist vaginal delivery at a level higher than this. Thus, the abdominal palpation component of this assessment is critical and decisive.

Other aspects of the vaginal assessment include recognising the sagittal suture and the occipital and parietal bones. The parietal bones always override the occipital bone, which is helpful in finding the posterior fontanelle. In this manner, the position and the degree of flexion of the fetal head can be defined. If the amount of caput makes this difficult then feel anteriorly for the fetal ear. Care should be taken to feel the pinna and the canal, as the ear can be folded and give a false impression of the true position. This landmark is also useful in assessing the level of the head and the likelihood of safe assisted delivery, because the ear is just below the maximum biparietal diameter. If it can be easily felt during maternal bearing-down effort, significant disproportion is unlikely. The assessment of caput and moulding is outlined in Chapter 2.

Synclitism is assessed by feeling the sagittal suture in its relationship to the transverse plane of the pelvic cavity. Anterior asynclitism, in which the anterior parietal bone is more easily felt and the sagittal suture further back in the transverse plane is normal. Posterior asynclitism is a sign of disproportion.

Clinical assessment of the bony pelvis has limitations but, with experience, it is useful in helping to define the relationship between this particular fetal head and bony pelvis. By measurement of one's own fingers, the obstetrician can assess the diagonal conjugate from the sacral promontory to beneath the pubic symphysis, the curve of the sacrum and the convergence of the pelvic sidewalls. The prominence of the ischial spines and sacrospinous ligaments can also be gauged. This, together with assessment of the fetal head: its position, station, degree of flexion or deflexion, asynclitism, caput, moulding, and the 'feel' of how this fits in the pelvis, is an important appraisal that, if carried out at every opportunity, will allow the obstetrician to gain the experience necessary to guide safe assisted vaginal delivery.

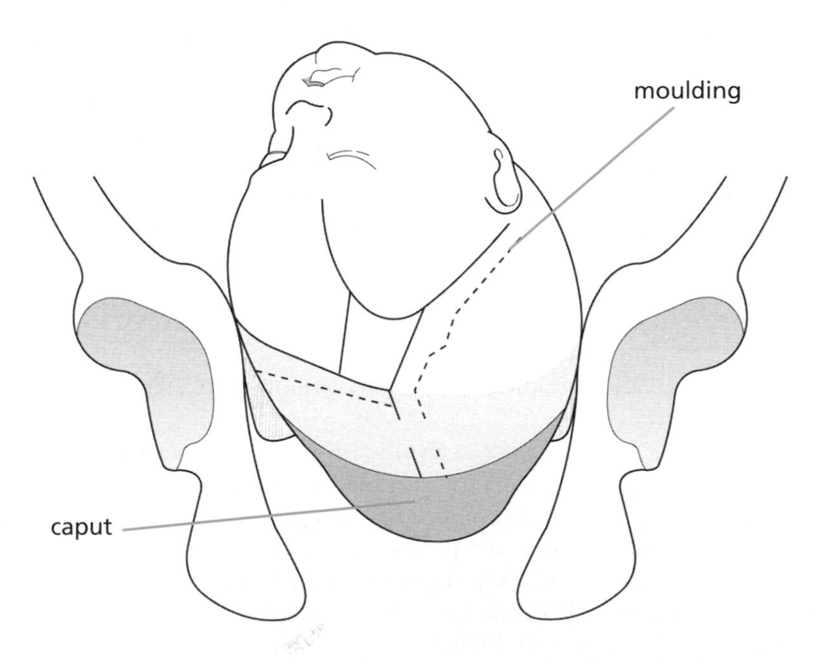

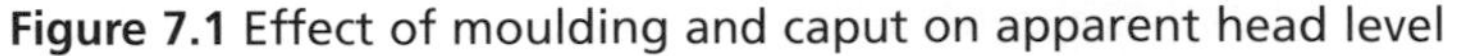
Figure 7.1 Effect of moulding and caput on apparent head level

ANALGESIA

Adequate analgesia may be provided in the form of epidural or spinal anaesthesia, pudendal block or local anaesthetic infiltration of the perineum. The amount required depends on the level of the fetal head and the need for rotation but, generally speaking, vacuum-assisted deliveries require less analgesia than forceps.

EMPTY THE BLADDER

This is best done by straight catheterisation just before carrying out the final combined abdominal/vaginal assessment.

TRIAL OF ASSISTED VAGINAL DELIVERY

In most cases it is clear that the head is in the low or outlet position and that assisted delivery will be accomplished with ease. However, in those cases in which the fetal head is arrested in between spines +1 to +2 cm it is often prudent to declare a trial of forceps or trial of vacuum. This entails an explanation to the woman and her partner, as well as the anaesthesia and nursing personnel, to the effect that she will be taken to the operating theatre where either assisted vaginal delivery or caesarean section can be performed. If the forceps or vacuum delivery proceeds smoothly, then vaginal delivery is safely achieved. However, if any difficulties are encountered the obstetrician can immediately back off and proceed to caesarean section. This declaration removes any pressure from the obstetrician to persist with an attempt at vaginal delivery when difficulty is encountered. It is a very important principle and often allows safe vaginal delivery of the fetus without increasing the risk (Revah *et al.* 1997).

Forceps delivery

About 700 different types of forceps have been described, although only some two-dozen are in common use. Broadly speaking, there are two types: classical forceps, used for direct traction, of which the most common are Simpson's forceps, and speciality forceps, used for rotation and traction (e.g. Kielland forceps) and for protection and flexion of the aftercoming head of the breech (Piper's forceps).

Before embarking upon forceps delivery, ensure that the conditions appropriate for assisted vaginal delivery outlined above have been fulfilled.

GENERAL CONSIDERATIONS

When appropriate time, oxytocin augmentation and maternal effort have been used and the fetal head has arrested at spines +1 cm to +3 cm, considerable skill and circumspection is required to avoid fetal and maternal trauma. Ironically, the well-flexed, occipitoanterior fetal head that has arrested at this level may be less favourable. In contrast to the deflexed occipitotransverse or occipitoposterior positions, which, when rotated to occipitoanterior will present a smaller diameter, the already well-flexed occipitoanterior head has arrested with the smallest diameter already presenting. Thus, the traction required to deliver the apparently favourable occipitoanterior position may be greater (Baskett 1997).

CLASSICAL FORCEPS

Delivery by this method is usually performed with the woman in the lithotomy position but outlet forceps can be applied with the woman in the left lateral position if the clinical situation demands.

The pelvic findings are carefully checked and the blades of the forceps assembled and well lubricated. The handle of the left blade is held in the left hand and applied to the left side of the fetal head. The blade is held parallel to the right inguinal ligament and inserted between the fetal head and the fingers, which protect the left posterolateral vaginal wall as the blade is inserted in a circular movement to negotiate the cephalic and pelvic curves. The right blade is inserted in a similar manner. The shanks and handles of the blades should sit horizontally: if one is at an angle and above the other blade, check for malposition or asynclitism. Slight inwards or downwards movements of the handles may be needed to 'snuggle' the blades into position. Correct application is ensured by noting that the sagittal suture is equidistant from the two blades and that there is equal space – about one fingerbreadth – between the fetal head and 'heel' of the blade. The powers of uterine contraction and maternal effort should be coordinated with steady traction downwards and backwards to negotiate the pelvic curve. Traction should not be carried out by gripping the handles but rather with the first and second fingers on the finger guards. The heel of the other hand may exert downward traction on the shanks (Pajot's manoeuvre) to ensure that traction is in the axis of the pelvic curve (Figure 7.2). As the head descends to the pelvic floor and begins to crown, the direction of pull arches upwards to gently deliver the head and face over the perineum. Episiotomy may be required at this stage. Some will remove the handles of the forceps at this point and assist final spontaneous delivery of the head over the perineum.

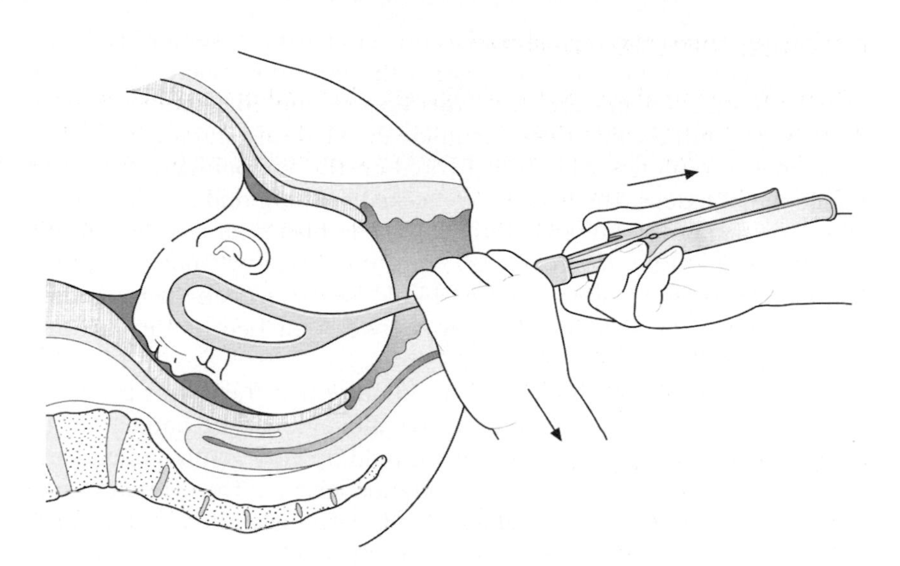

Figure 7.2 Pajot's manoeuvre

ROTATION FORCEPS

The most commonly used rotational forceps are those of Kielland. Considerable experience and skill are required for the safe use of this instrument (Tan *et al.* 1992). These forceps are designed for rotation of the head in the occipitotransverse or occipitoposterior position. As such, it has no pelvic curve, thus allowing rotation without maternal trauma. It also has a sliding lock to allow correction of asynclitism. By rotating the deflexed head to occipitoanterior and, in so doing, flexing it as well as correcting asynclitism, the narrowest diameter of the fetal head is presented to the pelvis.

The forceps are assembled and the directional knobs on the shanks face the occiput. The two common methods of application are direct and wandering techniques. In the direct technique, the anterior blade is applied under the symphysis at an angle that facilitates and guides the anterior blade over the curve of the fetal head. In the wandering technique, the anterior blade is applied in the traditional way along the lateral vaginal wall over the sinciput or face of the fetus and then gently 'wandered' under the symphysis pubis to lie on the side of the fetal head. In both techniques the posterior blade is applied directly. It is very important to insert the operator's hand in the posterior vagina as high as possible to protect the vaginal wall as one guides the posterior blade into position. As the tip of the blade passes the posterior aspect of the fetal head it is directed upward with the fingers and the handle directed downwards with the other hand to guide the blade around the fetal head. In a sense, the posterior blade is pivoted on the vaginal hand to protect the maternal tissues. The handles are locked together and the sliding lock allows correction of any asynclitism until the blades lie parallel and the handles lock easily together. As with the classical application, the relationship of the sagittal suture should be equidistant between the blades and about a fingerbreadth space between the heel of the blade and the fetal head.

Rotation of the head should be carried out when the uterus is relaxed and with a very gentle, slow progressive movement. The handles at the level of the junction with the shanks should be very gently grasped and depressed against the perineum as rotation occurs. Thus, rotation and flexion of the head should be achieved. It is extremely important to check that the head is rotating, as it is possible for the blades just to move around the fixed head. Under no circumstances should force be used for this manoeuvre – it is either achieved with a light touch or it is inappropriate to continue. It is at this stage that the cervical spine and cord are vulnerable (Menticoglou *et al.* 1995).

Once rotation and flexion of the fetal has occurred, the diameter of the fetal head presenting to the pelvis is reduced and can often be delivered with easy traction.

Vacuum extraction

The vacuum extractor is an alternative to forceps for assisted vaginal delivery and is gaining in popularity. It is associated with less trauma to the maternal pelvic floor and can usually be carried out with less anaesthesia.

Exactly the same safeguards apply to the use of the vacuum extractor as to the forceps. Since Malmström devised the first modern vacuum extractor in the early 1950s there have been a number of variations. Cups that have both the suction and traction points close to the middle are known as anterior cups. These are satisfactory if the head is occipitoanterior and well flexed. However, if the head is deflexed in the occipitotransverse or occipitoposterior position then the central vacuum port prevents the placement of the cup lateral enough to get it over the flexion point of the fetal head. This principle of the flexion point is central to the effective and safe application of the vacuum extractor (Bird 1976; Vacca 1992). In the term infant, the distance between the anterior and posterior fontanelles is approximately 9 cm. The flexion point is approximately 3 cm in front of the posterior fontanelle. Thus, when placing the centre of a 6-cm vacuum cup over the flexion point, the anterior edge of the cup will be approximately 3 cm behind the anterior fontanelle (Figure 7.3). If the cup is placed more anteriorly it will cause deflexion and therefore a larger diameter of the fetal head. If the cup is placed more to one side of the sagittal suture than the other, the application will be paramedian and present a larger diameter because of the asynclitism produced (Figure 7.4). The use of anterior cups to attempt delivery of deflexed occipitotransverse and occipitoposterior positions will often result in failure, as it is impossible to guide the cup over the flexion point because of the centrally placed vacuum ports. It is for this reason that it is essential to have a posterior cup, as originally designed by Bird, which, with the suction port placed peripherally allows manipulation of the cup laterally in the vagina over the flexion point of the occipitoposterior position. The principles of Bird's posterior cup have been incorporated into a new disposable rigid plastic device with an integral hand pump to create the vacuum – the OmniCup® (Clinical Innovations, Utah) (Vacca 2001).

Once the cup is properly applied the vacuum is created. A finger checks around the periphery of the cup to ensure that no maternal tissue is included. There is no advantage to the slow creation of the vacuum nor is it beneficial to reduce the vacuum between episodes of traction.

Traction should be applied at a right angle to the cup as much as possible to avoid the cup slipping ('pop-off'). During traction with the right hand, keep the left thumb on the top of the vacuum cup and the left index finger on the scalp. In this way, during traction one can see if the bony part of

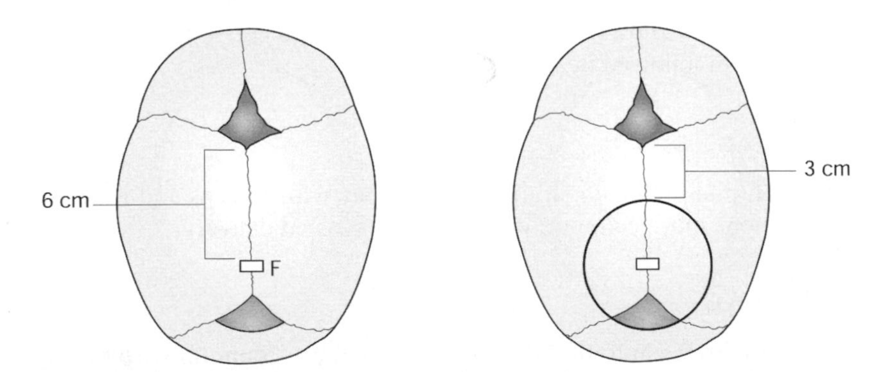

Figure 7.3 Defining the correct application of the vacuum cup over the flexion point

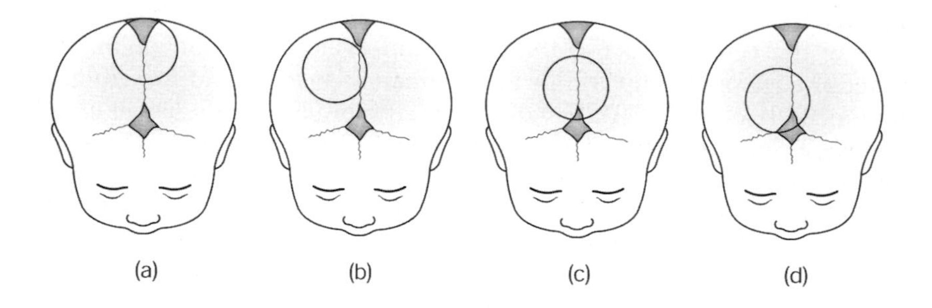

Figure 7.4 Correct and incorrect vacuum cup applications: (a) flexing median; (b) flexing paramedian; (c) deflexing median; (e) deflexing paramedian

the head is descending, rather than just the scalp. Traction is applied during a uterine contraction and aided by maternal effort. One 'pull' equals traction during one uterine contraction. As a general rule, a delivery should occur with three pulls or it should be clear that the head has descended to the perineum. It may take extra pulls to guide the head over the perineum. If the vacuum cup 'pops off', a very careful reappraisal should occur. One further application may be justified. Pop-offs are more common with soft cups but this does not make them less traumatic. Soft cups are also much more likely to fail to achieve delivery than the rigid, metal or plastic cups (O'Grady *et al.* 2000). If the cup pops off, consideration may be given to use forceps to complete delivery if the head is at the low/outlet level and very favourable. However, if there is failure to achieve delivery with the vacuum at the mid or low/mid level, only rarely should forceps be used to complete the delivery and caesarean section is usually chosen. The risk of fetal trauma is greatest with cases of failed vacuum followed by forceps delivery.

Complications

In general, maternal complications are higher with forceps and neonatal complications more common with vacuum assisted delivery.

MATERNAL

Vaginal lacerations and third degree tears are more common with forceps than vacuum delivery, although long-term pelvic floor function is similar in five-year follow up (Johanson *et al.* 1999).

FETAL

Superficial bruising and abrasions of the face and scalp are not uncommon with forceps but are usually trivial. Transient facial nerve palsy due to pressure on the seventh cranial nerve as it emerges from the stylomastoid foramen can occur. Serious cranial injuries such as depressed skull fracture and intracranial haemorrhage are rare. Cephalhaematoma is more common with vacuum than forceps but this is self-limiting and of no long-term clinical consequence. A rare but feared complication of vacuum delivery is subgaleal haemorrhage, in which blood vessels under the aponeurosis are disrupted and bleeding into this large area may result in lethal hypovolaemia. A large review showed that the rates of subdural or cerebral haemorrhage were similar in vacuum, forceps and caesarean delivery during labour (Towner *et al.* 1999). There is an increased incidence of retinal haemorrhage with vacuum extraction but no apparent adverse long-term sequelae.

Both the forceps and vacuum extractor have their place in modern obstetrics and the obstetrician should be familiar with the use of both instruments. As with all surgical manoeuvres, it is the judgement and skill of the person on the end of the instrument that dictates the outcome rather than the instrument itself.

For clinical audit and potential medico-legal purposes, it is essential that each assisted vaginal delivery be carefully documented immediately after delivery. This should include the indication, discussion of consent, a precise description of the station, moulding, caput, position and degree of flexion of the fetal head. A description of the procedure should follow with the manoeuvres, rotation, traction and level of difficulty. The number of 'pulls' (one pull equals traction during one uterine contraction) should be noted. Associated episiotomy or vaginal lacerations and their repair should be described.

References

ACOG. (2000) *Operative vaginal delivery: ACOG Practice Bulletin.* Washington DC: American College of Obstetricians and Gynecologists.

Baskett TF. (1997) Operative vaginal delivery in the 21st century. *J Soc Obstet Gynaecol Can* 19:355–7.

Bird GC. (1976) The importance of flexion in vacuum extraction delivery. *Br J Obstet Gynaecol* 83:194–200.

Bofill JA, Rust OA, Perry KG, Roberts WE, Martin RW, Morrison JC. (1996) Forceps and vacuum delivery: a survey of North American Residency Programs. *Obstet Gynecol* 88:622–5.

Drife JO. (1996) Choice and instrumental delivery. *Br J Obstet Gynaecol* 103:608–11.

Hankins GDV, Rowe TF. (1996) Operative vaginal delivery – year 2000. *Am J Obstet Gynecol* 175:275–82.

Hillier CEM, Johanson RB. (1994) Worldwide survey of assisted vaginal delivery. *Int J Gynaecol Obstet* 47:109–14.

Johanson RB, Heycock E, Carter J, Sultan AH, Walklate K, Jones PW. (1999) Maternal and child health after assisted vaginal delivery: five-year follow up of a randomised controlled study comparing forceps and Ventouse. *Br J Obstet Gynaecol* 106:544–9.

Knight D, Newnham JP, McKenna M, Evans S. (1993) A comparison of abdominal and vaginal examinations for the diagnosis of engagement of the fetal heart. *Aust N Z J Obstet Gynaecol* 33:154–8.

Menticoglou SM, Perlman M, Manning FA. (1995) High cervical spinal cord injury in neonates delivered with forceps: report of 15 cases. *Obstet Gynecol* 86:589–94.

O'Driscoll K, Meagher D, Boylan P. (1993) *Active Management of Labour*. 3rd ed. London: Mosby.

O'Grady JP, Pope CS, Patel SS. (2000) Vacuum extraction in modern obstetric practice: a review and critique. *Curr Opin Obstet Gynecol* 12:475–80.

Revah A, Ezra Y, Farine D, Ritchie K. (1997) Failed trial of vacuum or forceps: maternal and fetal outcome. *Am J Obstet Gynecol* 176:200–4.

RCOG. (2000). *Instrumental Vaginal Delivery. Guideline No. 26*. London: Royal College of Obstetricians and Gynaecologists.

Tan KH, Sim R, Yam KL. (1992) Kielland's forceps delivery: is it a dying art? *Singapore Med J* 33:380–2.

Towner D, Castro MA, Eby-Wilkens E, Gilbert WM. (1999) Effect of mode of delivery in nulliparous women on neonatal intracranial injury. *N Engl J Med* 341:1709–14.

Vacca A. (1992) *Handbook of Vacuum Extraction in Obstetric Practice*. Brisbane: Vacca Research.

Vacca A. (2001) Operative vaginal delivery: clinical appraisal of a new vacuum extraction device. *Aust N Z J Obstet Gynaecol* 41:156–60.

8 Breech vaginal delivery

The fetus presents by the breech in 3–4% of all deliveries, making it the most common malpresentation. Over the last 25 years, debate has continued as to whether the breech fetus is more safely delivered by caesarean section or assisted vaginal delivery (Cheng and Hannah 1993; Gifford *et al.* 1995; Danielian *et al.* 1996). In the interim, most obstetricians in developed countries have, as it were, voted with their scalpels, such that a steady increase in the proportion of breeches delivered by caesarean section has occurred. The debate has now been largely answered by the Canadian-organised international multicentre randomised trial (Hannah *et al.* 2000). Thus, where facilities exist, the standard of care will become elective caesarean section for breech presentation. Despite this intention to deliver all viable breech presentations by caesarean section, there will be occasions when vaginal delivery is unavoidable (Nwosu *et al.* 1993; SOGC 1994; ACOG 2001; RCOG 2001). Furthermore, the principles of atraumatic assisted vaginal breech delivery also apply to delivery of the breech through a uterine incision. It is for these reasons that we include this chapter on breech vaginal delivery.

The need for vaginal breech delivery may arise under the following circumstances:

- labour and delivery occur in a site where immediate caesarean section is not available
- the woman arrives at hospital in advanced labour with the breech already on the perineum
- incorrect diagnosis of the presenting part, such that a frank breech is mistaken for a cephalic presentation until late in the second stage of labour
- the woman may decide, even after being fully informed of the risks, that she wishes to proceed with vaginal delivery.

One of the problems with an almost universal policy of breech delivery by caesarean section is that it becomes a self-fulfilling prophecy that those in training will have inadequate exposure to assisted breech vaginal delivery. However, theoretical and practical training can be achieved using mannequins and, as mentioned above, most of the manoeuvres required for safe delivery of the breech through the uterine incision are similar to those required for assisted vaginal delivery (Baskett 1988). A disciplined and systematic approach to each case delivered by caesarean section can therefore help to provide the skills for those rare occasions when one is called upon to conduct a vaginal breech delivery.

In essence, the risks to the fetus in breech presentation are as follows:

- as a group, fetuses in breech presentation have a higher risk of intrinsic abnormalities than those with cephalic presentation. These may range from obvious anomalies to more subtle neurological abnormalities that may account for the overall worse outcome for breech infants, irrespective of the method of delivery
- asphyxia during labour is more common due to cord entanglement and/or prolapse
- intra-abdominal trauma due to excessive manipulation with the operator's hands encroaching on the fetal abdomen
- trauma to the fetal limbs, particularly in association with extended or nuchal arms.
- cervical spine injuries from excessive traction or torsion
- brachial plexus injuries from traction on the fetal body during attempts to deliver the head
- sudden decompression of the fetal head at the point of delivery causing tentorial tears and intracranial haemorrhage.

Management of breech delivery

The guiding principle is to allow the infant to deliver spontaneously with the minimum of intervention. However, a few specific points of assistance – particularly protective delivery of the head – are required to avoid some hazards.

FIRST STAGE OF LABOUR

If the first stage of labour is uneventful and progressive then a safe vaginal delivery is likely. Both the frank and complete types of breech are reasonable dilators of the cervix. Umbilical cord compression due to entanglement or prolapse is more common and should be routinely excluded by pelvic examination after rupture of the membranes or if there is abnormality of the fetal heart rate. One of the great potential hazards is due to the fact that the breech and trunk of the fetus is smaller in diameter than the aftercoming head. This is even more exaggerated in the premature infant. Thus, it is possible for the breech and legs to appear at the introitus through an incompletely dilated cervix. If delivery is attempted, the dreaded complication of entrapment of the fetal head by an incompletely dilated cervix is realised. It is essential, therefore, in all cases to ensure that the cervix is fully dilated and retracted before proceeding with delivery.

ANAESTHESIA

In many instances, provided that it gives the woman adequate analgesia, the combination of narcotic, inhalation and pudendal block analgesia allows the most natural progression of the first and second stages of labour. However, there is much to be gained with epidural analgesia, particularly in preventing premature maternal bearing-down effort in the late first and early second stages of labour before the cervix has fully dilated and completely retracted into the lower uterine segment. On the other hand, one wants full maternal effort during the second stage, so a selective type of epidural that allows retention of motor function is the ideal. An anaesthetist should be present at all breech deliveries for the rare case when rapid general anaesthesia or uterine relaxation is required.

DELIVERY OF THE BREECH AND LEGS

The key point is 'Hands off the breech'. In general, manoeuvres involving rotation and flexion of the limbs and trunk are helpful and those involving traction are not. The breech should be allowed to descend to the perineum with maternal effort alone. At this point, the patient can be placed in the lithotomy position and, if appropriate, a pudendal block performed, together with local anaesthetic infiltration of the perineum. As the breech meets the opposition of the perineum the anterior buttock 'climbs up' the fourchette. Once the anterior buttock ascends to the point where the fetal anus is visible over the fourchette (this is usually heralded by a bead of meconium) the point has been reached when further spontaneous progression will only occur when the obstruction of the perineum has been removed by a generous mediolateral episiotomy. In a footling breech, the point at which episiotomy should be performed is when the buttocks reach the perineum. In a multiparous woman with a lax perineum an episiotomy may not be necessary.

Wait until the beginning of a contraction before performing the episiotomy. This will allow maternal effort during one entire uterine contraction to help deliver the buttocks and legs. Here again it is appropriate to keep your hands off the breech and allow spontaneous progression. Only if it is a frank breech with extended legs will assistance be necessary in the form of two fingers placed behind the fetal thigh to flex the hip and knee and allow delivery of the leg. This is done for each leg in turn. The remainder of the fetal abdomen and lower trunk will then follow by maternal effort alone. Check that the umbilical cord is not under undue tension and, if it is, gently hook down a loop of cord. The fetal back will usually remain anterolateral during this time. If the back shows any tendency to rotate posteriorly it should be gently guided to the anterior position. It is very important not to put traction on the fetus at this point, as this will serve only to extend the fetal arms and head. This requires discipline, as one instinctively wants to aid the process of delivery. So, other than the few manoeuvres required above, continue to 'keep your hands off the breech'.

DELIVERY OF THE SHOULDERS AND ARMS

With maternal effort alone, the remainder of the trunk should be expelled and the lower border of one scapula will become visible under the pubic arch.

The fetal head is now entering the pelvic brim and the umbilical cord will be partially or completely occluded. One should note the time on the clock and plan to have the delivery complete within the next two to three minutes. This is when fine judgement is required to run the gauntlet between excessive haste and potentially traumatic delivery and waiting too long so that hypoxia will supervene.

Once the scapula is visible, the arms will probably be flexed in front of the fetus. Their delivery, if not spontaneous, can easily be achieved by passing the index and middle fingers over the shoulder and then splinting and sweeping the humerus down across the chest. The fetal back is rotated 90 degrees to bring the other scapula into view and the procedure repeated on the other arm.

For rotation of the fetal back or other manoeuvres required to deliver extended arms (see below), appropriate placement of the operator's hands is important. The instinct is to grasp the infant around the hips and abdomen. This is potentially traumatic to the intra-abdominal contents. The hands must be placed lower than this – around the thighs and hips of the fetus, so that the thumbs are on the sacrum and the upper fingers around the iliac crest. A small sterile towel will help maintain the grip during this manoeuvre.

EXTENDED ARMS

When extended arms occur, it is usually because inappropriate traction has been placed on the fetus before this point. Løvset's manoeuvre is an effective way of dealing with this complication. It is based on the principle that the posterior fetal shoulder enters the maternal pelvic cavity before the anterior shoulder. In the manner mentioned above, the fetal thighs and hips are grasped and the body lifted anteriorly to cause lateral flexion and promote descent of the posterior shoulder below the sacral promontory. The fetal back is kept uppermost, as the body is rotated 180 degrees so that the posterior shoulder (below the pelvic brim) is now rotated to become the anterior shoulder. As such, it is now below the symphysis and the humerus can be hooked down with ease. The body is then rotated back through 180 degrees, which brings the other shoulder below the symphysis and allows delivery of that arm (Figure 8.1).

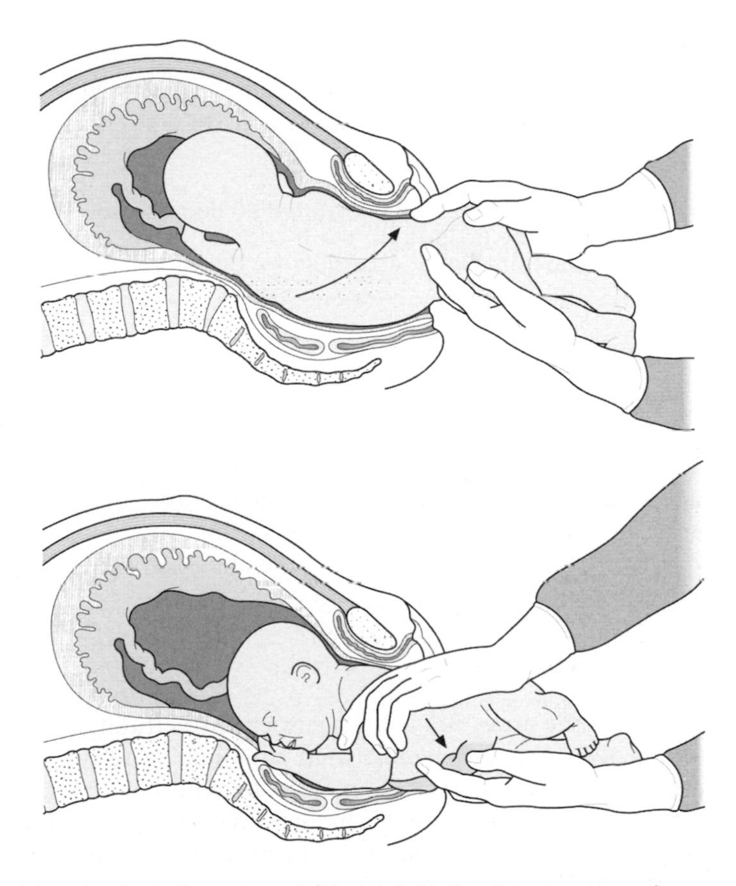

Figure 8.1 Lovset's manoeuvre: (a) lateral flexion is exaggerated to facilitate descent of the posterior shoulder beneath the promontory; with the back upper most, the body is rotated 180 degrees; (b) the posterior shoulder has now been rotated anteriorly beneath the symphysis and can be hooked down; the body is then rotated 180 degrees and the other arm delivered in the same way

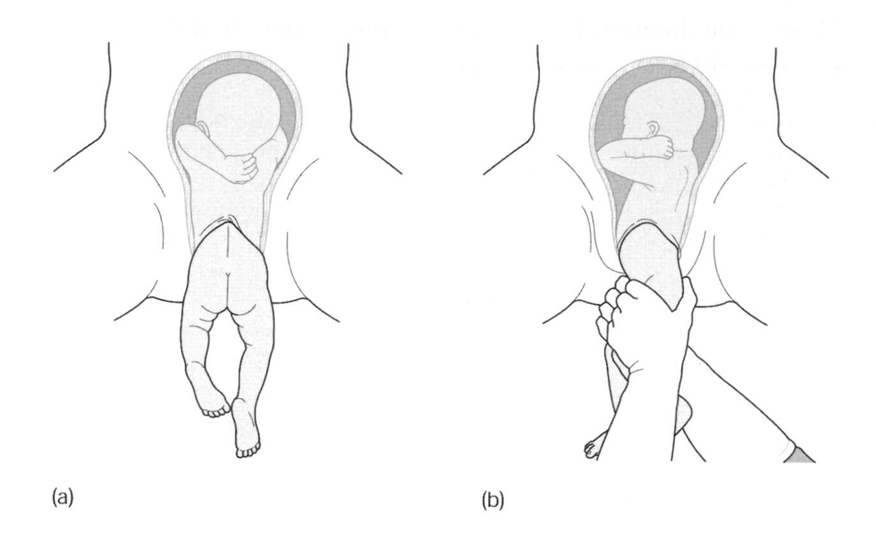

Figure 8.2 Nuchal arm: (a) the body is rotated 90 degrees freeing the forearm from behind the occiput; (b) the friction of rotation promotes flexion of the shoulder making it accessible for delivery

NUCHAL ARM

In this situation, the shoulder is extended and the elbow flexed so that the forearm is trapped behind the occiput. This usually occurs because of inappropriate traction and rotational manoeuvres at an earlier stage in the delivery. To overcome this problem, the fetal trunk is rotated in the direction of the fetal hand (Figure 8.2). The occiput thus rotates past the arm and, with further rotation, flexion of the shoulder should occur and allow delivery of the arm.

DELIVERY OF THE HEAD

After delivery of the arms, the baby is suspended vertically with partial support from the operator's hands. Mild suprapubic pressure from an assistant may help descent and flexion of the fetal head. The baby should not be allowed to hang entirely by its own weight as this may, paradoxically, promote extension of the head. Once the hairline on the fetal neck is visible beneath the pubic arch, the head is ready for assisted delivery. Assistance at this stage is necessary to avoid the sudden decompression of the perineum on the fetal head at the point of delivery. This 'champagne cork' delivery can lead to tentorial tears and intracranial haemorrhage. For this reason, the head must be controlled at delivery in all cases and there are two main techniques to achieve this:

- forceps to the aftercoming head
- Mauriceau–Smellie–Veit manoeuvre.

Forceps to the aftercoming head

This is usually the best method and provides the most efficient protection and controlled delivery of the fetal head. An additional asset of forceps is that they encourage flexion of the head and are the safest way to apply the mild traction that may be necessary to complete delivery.

While an assistant holds the fetal body just above the horizontal plane the forceps are applied below the body at the four and eight o'clock positions along the sides of the fetal head (Figure 8.3). Most of the long-handled forceps can be used but Piper's forceps were especially developed for this purpose as they have a long shank. At this stage it is important not to allow the fetal body to be raised much above the horizontal, as this risks hyperextension of and trauma to the fetal cervical spine. As the head is delivering, and once the fetal chin and mouth are visible, the forceps and the body of the fetus are raised together to complete delivery.

Mauriceau–Smellie–Veit manoeuvre

This method does not provide quite the same degree of protection and control as forceps. However, it can be useful when events happen so rapidly that application of forceps is not feasible. The operator's forearm is placed under the fetal body so that it lies astride the forearm. The forefinger and middle fingers are placed on the maxilla beside the nose

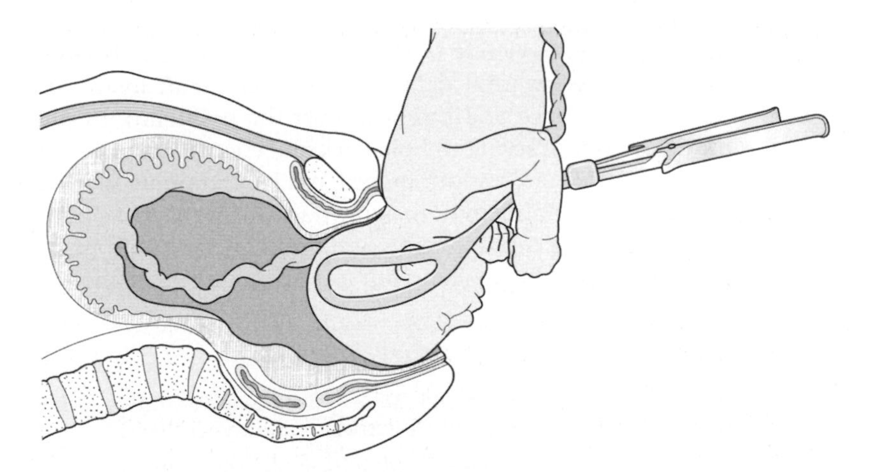

Figure 8.3 Forceps to the aftercoming head

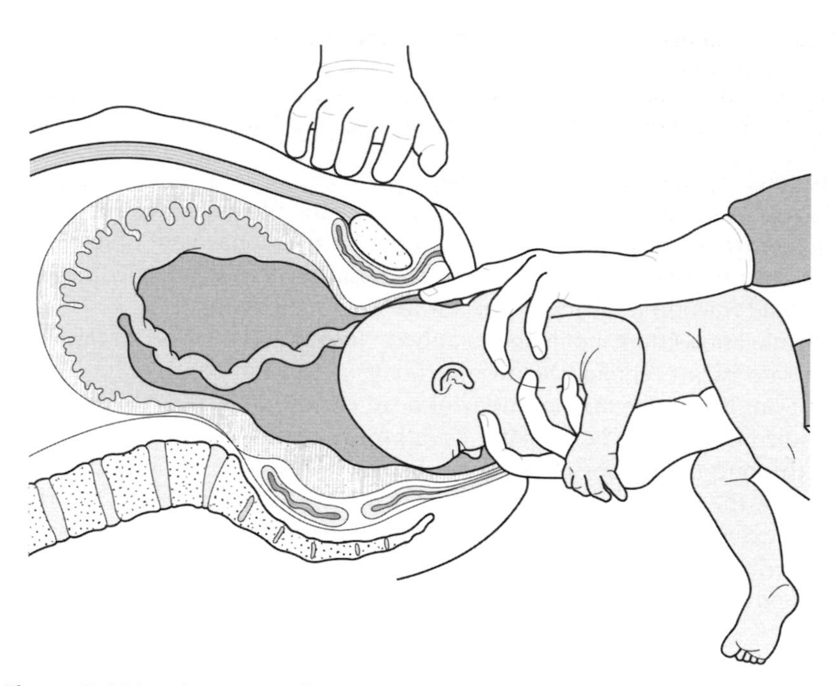

Figure 8.4 Mauriceau–Smellie–Veit manoeuvre

and promote flexion of the fetal head. The other hand is placed on the fetal back, the middle finger pushing upwards on the occiput also to enhance flexion of the head, while the other fingers are resting on the fetal shoulders (Figure 8.4). Gentle traction in a downward and backward direction may be necessary until delivery of the fetal chin followed by upward guidance of the face and forehead over the perineum. In many cases, it is more a matter of trying to hold back and control delivery of the head to avoid sudden decompression. Indeed, it is inappropriate to use the Mauriceau–Smellie–Veit manoeuvre to apply traction, as this risks trauma to the brachial plexus and cervical spine. If more than very mild traction is needed then this should be applied with forceps as described above.

References

ACOG. (2001) *Committee Opinion No 265. Mode of Term Singleton Breech Delivery.* Washington DC: American College of Obstetricians and Gynecologists.

Baskett TF. (1988) Trends in operative obstetrical delivery: implications for specialist training. *Ann R Coll Physicians Surg Can* 1988;1:1119–21.

Cheng M, Hannah M. (1993) Breech delivery at term: a critical review of the literature. *Obstet Gynecol*;82:605–18.

Danielian PJ, Wang J, Hall MH. (1996) Long-term outcome by method of delivery of fetuses in breech presentation at term: population-based follow-up. *BMJ* 312:1451–3.

Gifford DS, Morton SC, Fiske M. (1995) A meta-analysis of infant outcomes after breech delivery. *Obstet Gynecol* 85:1047–54.

Hannah ME, Hannah WJ, Hewson SA, Hodnett ED, Saigal S, Willan AR. (2000) Planned caesarean section versus planned vaginal birth for breech presentation at term: a randomised multicentre trial. *Lancet* 356:1375–83.

Nwosu EC, Walkinshaw S, Chia P, Manasse PR, Atlay RD. (1993) Undiagnosed breech. *Br J Obstet Gynaecol* 100:531–5.

RCOG. (2001) *The Management of Breech Presentation. Guideline No 20.* London: Royal College of Obstetricians and Gynaecologists.

SOGC (Society of Obstetricians and Gynaecologists of Canada). Canadian Consensus on Breech Management at Term. (1994) *J Soc Obstet Gynaecol Can* 16:1839–48.

9 Twin and triplet delivery

Over the past 25 years, due to assisted reproductive technology, the incidence of multiple pregnancy has increased from 1.0 to 1.5% of all maternities in many developed countries (Joseph *et al.* 1998). Compared with singleton pregnancies, the perinatal morbidity and mortality of twins is increased five- to ten-fold and much more for triplets and higher-order multiple births. For example: compared with singletons, cerebral palsy is increased eight-fold in twins and about 40-fold with triplets (Petterson *et al.* 1993; Yokoyama *et al.*1995). The main determinants of this increase in morbidity and mortality are prematurity, growth restriction, anomalies and twin-to-twin transfusion. Asphyxia and trauma during delivery make a smaller contribution to morbidity and mortality but can be all the more tragic when the safe conclusion of a high-risk pregnancy is at hand. It is therefore understandable that in many developed countries the caesarean section rate for twins has roughly doubled, from 25% to 50%, over the last 25 years, although there is no proof that abdominal delivery is safer for the infants. It is clear, however, that irrespective of the mode of delivery, twins should be supervised in hospitals with adequate anaesthetic, obstetric and neonatal personnel and facilities.

Obstetric factors

At the time of delivery the most common presentations in twin pregnancies are (twin A/twin B):

- vertex/vertex
- vertex/breech
- breech/vertex
- breech/breech.

This covers more than 90% of the combinations, with the remainder involving transverse lie of one or both fetuses. In practical terms, the most common combinations are:

- vertex/vertex 40%
- vertex/non-vertex 35–40%
- non-vertex/other 20–25%.

Thus, in 75–80% of cases, the first twin is in cephalic presentation and this will be the dominant factor in the decision to allow labour and vaginal delivery. There are those who feel that if the second twin is in a non-vertex position at the start of labour this justifies caesarean section. However, in about 20% of cases the position of the second twin will change after delivery of the first and may go from an unfavourable to a favourable position or, alternatively, from a favourable to an unfavourable lie. In addition, the option is available for version of the second twin should it be in an unfavourable presentation or, in extreme cases, to deliver the second twin by caesarean section. Thus, the lie or presentation of the second twin at the start of labour should not influence the decision to allow labour and vaginal delivery.

Individual factors, however, will influence the decision for or against labour and vaginal delivery. This will include the availability of appropriate facilities and personnel. Clinical factors to be evaluated include:

- extremes of estimated fetal weight (less than 1500 g, greater than 3500 g)
- weight discrepancy between twins A and B (particularly if twin B is larger than twin A)
- potential fetal compromise from growth restriction or twin-to-twin transfusion.

Monochorionic, monoamniotic placentation only accounts for 1% of all twins but the risk of cord and fetal entanglement is such that all should be delivered by elective caesarean section. Maternal considerations will include age, parity, history of infertility and previous obstetric factors such as caesarean section.

The second twin faces potential increased risks during labour. After the first twin has been delivered, the reduction in uterine size or partial placental separation may reduce blood flow to the intervillous space creating hypoxia. There is also a greater risk of trauma to the second twin due to intrauterine manipulations required for malpresentation.

Anaesthetic factors

There is much in favour of epidural analgesia for twin delivery. If epidural is unavailable, pudendal block and local infiltration of the perineum performed just before delivery of the first twin should allow most of the vaginal manipulations required to deliver the second twin.

Epidural is the ideal, as it will allow both vaginal and intrauterine manipulations and cover the unlikely need to deliver the second twin by caesarean section. The limitation of epidural anaesthesia is the fact that it does not cause uterine relaxation. This is of critical importance if delivery of the second twin by internal version and breech extraction is undertaken. In these cases, the choice is either to superimpose general anaesthesia on top of the epidural or provide short-term uterine relaxation with intravenous glyceryl trinitrate. The latter is more acceptable. This is one of a number of uses for emergency short-term uterine relaxation with glyceryl trinitrate and the details of administration will be covered here (Baskett 1999).

Glyceryl trinitrate comes in an ampoule containing 5 mg in 1 ml. A reasonable approach is to dilute this 1 ml (5 mg) in a 100-ml bag of physiological saline. This produces a solution of 50 μg/per ml. If 20 ml of this solution is drawn into a syringe it allows one to give accurate doses of 50 μg/per ml. Given intravenously, glyceryl trinitrate rapidly achieves a high concentration and is equally rapidly degraded in one to three minutes. Thus, it is possible to titrate a fairly precise and safe response. Peripheral vasodilatation and reduced venous tone may cause significant maternal hypotension, so it is important to ensure that the woman is not hypovolaemic when giving this drug. This vasodilatation responds to ephedrine and the uterine relaxation responds to oxytocin (Lau *et al.* 2001). It is usual to start with a dose of 200 μg and repeat this at one- to two-minute intervals until adequate uterine relaxation is achieved. Obstetric anaesthetists and obstetricians must be aware of the need for complete uterine relaxation in order to safely carry out internal version and breech extraction for the second twin.

Management of labour

FIRST STAGE OF LABOUR

The first stage of labour is managed as for a singleton fetus. If the first twin is other than a vertex presentation it will probably be delivered by elective caesarean section. If possible, both twins should have fetal heart rate monitoring during labour. Oxytocin induction and/or augmentation of labour with twins is acceptable if indicated. An intravenous infusion should be established and epidural anaesthesia provided as required. Spontaneous or assisted vaginal delivery of the first twin involves the same principles as for a singleton fetus. Additional obstetric and neonatal personnel should be alerted with the anticipation of immediate neonatal care for both twins (Benachi and Pons 1998).

SECOND STAGE OF LABOUR

Many prefer to conduct the second stage in a room where there is the capability of moving straight to caesarean section for those rare cases in which this is needed for the second twin. The availability of ultrasound may help define the lie and presentation of the second twin when there is clinical doubt.

When the first twin delivers, its cord should be securely clamped in case there is a vascular connection that would allow the second twin to bleed through the cord of the first. After delivery of the first twin there is usually a reduction in uterine contractions. Thus, it is advisable at this time to set-up an intravenous infusion with 5 units of oxytocin in 500 ml crystalloid 'piggy-backed' on to the main intravenous line. As in much of intrapartum care, good judgement is required to achieve a balance between excessive intervention leading to hurried and traumatic delivery and passive delay, which might end with asphyxia. This endeavour is aided by careful fetal heart rate monitoring of the second twin.

GUIDELINES FOR DELIVERING THE SECOND TWIN

- Once the first twin has been delivered check the lie and presentation of the second twin. If the presentation is cephalic or breech, this pole is steadied at the pelvic brim with one hand while a pelvic examination rules out cord presentation. The 'piggy-backed' oxytocin infusion is started at about ten drops per minute and, when contractions are regular and the presenting part stable and descending, the membranes are ruptured. Usually the fetus will descend with a few contractions to spontaneous or assisted delivery.
- If the second twin is a transverse or oblique lie then external cephalic or podalic version should convert the lie to longitudinal and allow one to proceed as above.
- If the second twin is a footling breech or transverse lie and, particularly if the transverse lie does not respond to external version, a case can be made for immediate internal version and/or breech extraction. This is one of the few valid indications for these procedures in modern obstetrics. As mentioned in the section on anaesthetic factors, it is essential for the uterus to be well relaxed before these manoeuvres are considered. A well-relaxed uterus, together with the recent passage of the first twin, creates ideal conditions for this form of delivery.

TECHNICAL ASPECTS OF INTERNAL VERSION AND BREECH EXTRACTION

- With appropriate anaesthesia and uterine relaxation, the forewaters should not be tense and you will be able to feel the parts of the fetus.
- Keeping the membranes intact, grasp one or preferably both feet and pull steadily downwards and backwards into the vagina.
- The relaxed uterus and cushion of amniotic fluid ensure that the fetus converts readily from transverse to breech.
- As you continue traction, the membranes will rupture, but by this stage the breech is well on its way to the introitus, having being buffered from trauma by the amniotic fluid during its descent.
- Continue traction until the scapula appears.
- Carry out the remainder of the delivery as outlined in the chapter on breech vaginal delivery.

When reaching through the membranes for the foot, it is obviously important not to confuse this with the hand. The foot is best identified by the point of the heel. One can practice this by feeling the hands and feet of newborn infants with one's eyes closed during other normal births. It is preferable to grasp both feet, but if only one can be reached it is better that it is the anterior foot. If one has grasped the posterior foot, the anterior buttock may arrest on the pubic symphysis during traction. If this occurs the posterior leg should be rotated 180 degrees in a wide arc during traction to convert it to the anterior position. In these cases, the second leg will be extended and can be brought down in the same manner as the extended leg of a frank breech.

If there is intrapartum bleeding, cord prolapse, a non-reassuring fetal heart rate pattern, or continued delay despite oxytocin augmentation, then delivery should be accelerated. The options include assisted vaginal delivery with forceps or vacuum for cephalic presentations, breech extraction or caesarean section (Persad *et al.* 2001). The choice will depend upon the available facilities, anaesthesia, experience of the attendant and the lie and station of the second twin.

An outline of the intrapartum management of the most common combinations in twin pregnancy is shown in Figure 9.1.

LOCKED TWINS

Locked twins are extremely rare, occurring in about one per thousand

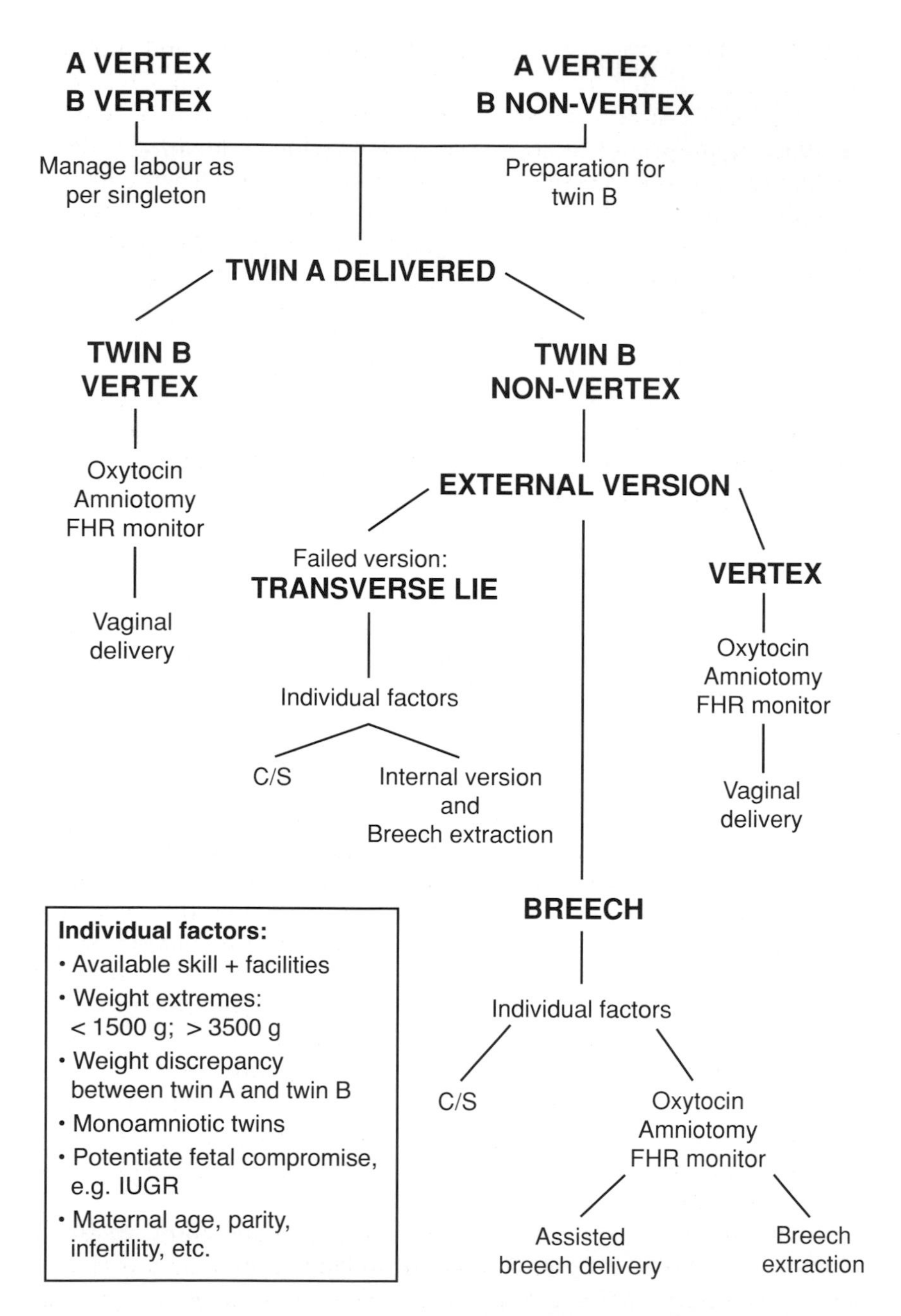

Figure 9.1 Intrapartum management of twin pregnancy; C/S = caesarean section; FHR = fetal heart rate; IUGR = intrauterine growth restriction

(reproduced from Baskett TF. Essential Management of Obstetric Emergencies. 3rd ed. 1999, with permission of Clinical Press Ltd.)

twin deliveries. However, the risk of lethal asphyxia and trauma, particularly to the first twin, is high. The most likely occurrence is with relatively small fetuses when twin A is breech and twin B vertex. In most obstetric units nowadays twins with this presentation at the start of labour would undergo caesarean section. When locked twins are encountered, it is usual for the first twin breech to deliver normally up to the trunk but the delivery of the shoulders and descent of the arms and head is arrested. On occasions, under deep general anaesthesia with uterine relaxation, one can elevate the body of the first twin and disimpact the head of the second twin. This allows one to proceed with breech delivery of the first twin and deal with the second in the usual manner. If, however, gentle attempts at disimpaction fail, then one is usually committed to delivery by caesarean section. This will entail a generous classical incision in the uterus to allow 'reverse extraction' of the first twin through the uterine incision, followed by the second twin.

Third stage of labour

After delivery of twins, the overdistended uterus is more prone to atony. Thus, active management of the third stage of labour should be followed by an extended (six- to eight-hour) intravenous infusion of oxytocin.

Triplets and higher-order births

With the use of ovulation-induction agents and assisted reproduction techniques, triplets and higher-order births have increased three-fold in many developed countries. In many units the majority, if not all, viable triplets are delivered by elective caesarean section. In addition to obviating the need for experienced and skilled intrauterine and vaginal manipulation, another advantage is that of allowing the scheduling of three teams for immediate neonatal care. It is also difficult to monitor the fetal hearts of triplets in labour. However, the risks of caesarean section to the mother are greater and there is no evidence that there is clear benefit to the infants from abdominal versus vaginal delivery. Indeed, it has been suggested that vaginal delivery of triplets at 32–34 weeks of gestation may hold some advantages for the infant (Dommergues *et al.* 1995, 1998; Wildshut *et al.* 1995).

Vaginal delivery may be considered in selected cases at 32 weeks of gestation and above, with the first triplet in cephalic presentation and no signs of fetal compromise in any of the triplets. Once the first triplet has been born the next two should be delivered without delay. If they present by the vertex, the membranes can be ruptured and spontaneous or low assisted delivery carried out. If not, immediate internal version and/or breech extraction, with the same safeguards as outlined for the second twin, should be undertaken.

For quadruplets and above planned caesarean section will be chosen for viable pregnancies.

References

Baskett TF. (1999) Emergency uterine relaxation. In: *Essential Management of Obstetric Emergencies*. 3rd ed. Bristol: Clinical Press. p. 110–14.

Benachi A, Pons JC. (1998) Is the route of delivery a meaningful issue in twins? *Clin Obstet Gynecol* 41:31–5.

Dommergues M, Mahieu-Caputo D, Mandelbrot L, Huon C, Moriette C, Dumez Y. (1995) Delivery of uncomplicated triplet pregnancies: is the vaginal route safer? A case–control study. *Am J Obstet Gynecol* 172:513–7.

Dommergues M, Mahieu-Caputo D, Dumez Y. (1998) Is the route of delivery a meaningful issue in triplets and higher order multiples? *Clin Obstet Gynecol* 41:25–9.

Joseph KS, Kramer MS, Marcoux S, Ohlsson A, Wen SW, Allen A, Platt R. (1998) Determinants of preterm birth in Canada from 1981 through 1983 and 1992 through 1994. *N Engl J Med* 339:1434–9.

Lau LC, Adaikau PG, Arulkumaran S, Ng SC. (2001) Oxytocics reverse the tocolytic effect of glyceryl trinitrate on the human uterus. *Br J Obstet Gynaecol* 108:164–8.

Persad VL, Baskett TF, O'Connell CM, Scott HM. (2001) Combined vaginal-cesarean delivery of twin pregnancies. *Obstet Gynecol* 98:1032–7.

Petterson B, Nelson KB, Watson L, Stanley F. (1993) Twins, triplets, and cerebral palsy in births in Western Australia in the 1980s. *BMJ* 307:1239–43.

Wildshut HIJ, Van Roosmalen J, Van Leeuwen E, Keirse MJNC. (1995) Planned abdominal compared with planned vaginal birth in triplet pregnancies. *Br J Obstet Gynaecol* 102:292–6.

Yokoyama Y, Shimizu T, Hayakawa K. (1995) Prevalence of cerebral palsy in twins, triplets, and quadruplets. *Int J Epidemiol* 24:943–8.

10 Caesarean section

Over the last quarter of the 20th century, caesarean section rates increased worldwide, making it the most common operation in obstetrics and gynaecology. A variety of factors have lowered the threshold for performing caesarean section (Savage 2000; Drife and Walker 2001; Guihard and Blondel 2001).

- Improvements in anaesthesia, blood transfusion, antibiotics, surgical techniques and thromboprophylaxis have combined to increase the safety of caesarean section.
- There is now a combination of social and medico-legal expectations of perfection in perinatal outcome.
- Less experience and an unwillingness to accept even small increased risks associated with certain types of operative vaginal delivery. Even before the recent randomised trial showed that caesarean section was safer than vaginal delivery for term breech presentation, a majority of obstetricians had anticipated the results and shunned the vaginal route (Hannah *et al* 2000).
- Increasing maternal age, infertility and assisted reproductive technologies have led to a rise in the number of so-called 'premium' pregnancies.
- Improved neonatal care and outcome has lowered the gestational age at which caesarean section is appropriate for fetal indications.
- A rare but potentially emerging indication is women requesting elective caesarean section for the perceived benefits of eliminating rare fetal risks in labour and the sequelae of pelvic floor damage to themselves (Paterson-Brown and Amu 1998).

Indications

While the indications and their proportion may vary from country to country and hospital to hospital, the big four indications account for 60–90% of all caesarean sections:

- repeat caesarean section (35–40%)

- dystocia (20–35%)
- breech (10–15%)
- fetal distress (10–15%).

In many cases there is a combination of dystocia and fetal distress in a non-progressive labour associated with a non-reassuring fetal heart rate pattern. These indications are discussed in their respective chapters.

General considerations

ANAESTHESIA

Anaesthesia for caesarean section should be regional (epidural or spinal) in the vast majority of cases. Exceptions requiring general anaesthesia will be:

- patient preference (rare)
- need for speed (acute fetal distress)
- possibility of prolonged surgery, such as uterine rupture or placenta praevia accreta.

PROPHYLACTIC ANTIBIOTICS

Prophylactic antibiotics are indicated in all but elective caesarean sections with intact membranes (Hopkins and Smaill 2000). Some obstetricians will give an antibiotic to all mothers delivering by caesarean section in an attempt to minimise febrile morbidity. A single intravenous dose, given at cord clamping, of a first-generation broad-spectrum antibiotic such as ampicillin or cephalosporin is effective. In cases with risk factors, such as prolonged labour with ruptured membranes or when there are clinical signs of early chorioamnionitis, the antibiotic may be continued for 24–48 hours.

THROMBOPROPHYLAXIS

Thromboprophylaxis with compression leg stockings and low-dose subcutaneous heparin is indicated with risk factors (RCOG 1995).

Types of caesarean section

LOWER TRANSVERSE SEGMENT CAESAREAN SECTION

Lower transverse segment caesarean section is the type of operation performed in about 98% of cases. The uterine incision is confined to the relatively non-contractile lower uterine segment so that its healing is optimal and potential disruption less likely in a subsequent labour.

LOW VERTICAL CAESAREAN SECTION

Low vertical caesarean section has been advocated by some, when the lower segment is well developed by advanced labour but, because of earlier gestational age, the width of the lower segment is deemed inadequate to deliver the fetus atraumatically through a transverse incision. This incision also obviates the risk of trauma to the uterine vessels. Should the incision require enlargement it can be extended vertically into the upper uterine segment to achieve delivery of the fetus. In fact, many so-called low vertical incisions do extend into the upper uterine segment and have at least some of the drawbacks to the classical incision. Thus, this type of incision is rarely performed and usually only by enthusiastic advocates.

CLASSICAL CAESAREAN SECTION

Classical caesarean section will comprise 1–2% of all caesarean sections in most obstetric units. This rate has increased as the gestational age at which caesarean section is performed has fallen (Bethune and Permezel 1997). The vertical incision in the upper uterine segment has the disadvantage of being more vascular and the healing in the puerperium may be disrupted in this contractile portion of the uterus. As outlined in Chapter 11, the subsequent rupture of this scar in another pregnancy carries a much higher risk. The most common indication is caesarean section in the earlier weeks of gestation when inadequate formation of the lower uterine segment precludes safe and atraumatic delivery of the fetus through that site. It is also necessary when access to the lower uterine segment is prohibited by uterine fibroids, extensive adhesions, or the massive vascularity rarely associated with some cases of major placenta praevia.

In the vast majority of cases, a lower transverse incision can be planned and performed. In patients of earlier gestation, particularly below 34 weeks, and if there has been no labour, the lower segment may not be adequately formed to allow delivery of the fetus through an incision in that site. The final decision can only be taken when the abdomen is opened and the lower segment is inspected directly. As the advantages of the lower transverse incision are considerable, in some marginal cases one starts with this incision but accepts, if there is difficulty in delivering the fetus, that an additional vertical incision, either a 'J' extension into the upper segment on one side, or the inverted 'T' in the midline, may have to be performed (Boyle and Gabbe 1996). In many such cases one can safely perform the lower transverse incision and save the woman the subsequent risks of a classical incision. In those women in whom one has to resort to the 'J' or inverted 'T' incision, the end result is no worse than a classical incision.

Surgical aspects

LOWER TRANSVERSE SEGMENT CAESAREAN SECTION

As with all operations, individual surgeons develop their own points of technique (Tully *et al.* 2002). However, the following general guidelines seem reasonable.

- To avoid aortocaval compression by the uterus the woman is placed with a lateral tilt of 15 degrees.
- In the majority of all types of caesarean section the Pfannenstiel incision or modification thereof is adequate and appropriate (Stark and Finkel 1994; Darj and Nordstrom 1999). The main indication for a lower midline incision is speed of entry for acute fetal compromise or in cases where both speed and extra surgical space may be required, such as uterine rupture.
- A urethral Foley catheter should be inserted preoperatively and may be retained for a few hours or overnight following the procedure. During labour the bladder is elevated and unless it is empty it is even more vulnerable to incision during entry to the peritoneal cavity. For this reason, the peritoneum is first incised as high as possible and extended down under transillumination.
- Once the peritoneal cavity has been opened, check the uterus for dextro- or laevo-rotation. It is more common to find dextro-rotation due to the sigmoid colon. This has important implications for placement of the incision in the uterus. If this point is ignored, it is easy to make the transverse incision in an eccentric manner such that the uterine vessels are breached on one side.

  The uterovesical peritoneum is identified and incised and, with the forefinger, the areolar tissue between the lower uterine segment and bladder gently separated. A Doyen, DeLee or Balfour retractor is then placed to move the bladder down safely from the line of uterine incision.
- Be aware that in prolonged labour with disproportion the lower uterine segment may be stretched and drawn up to form a considerable portion of the lower uterus. In such cases, if the uterine incision is made too low, one risks entering the vagina. Careful attention to the point of reflection from the uterus of the uterovesical peritoneal fold will help with the appropriate placement of the uterine incision.

The initial incision into the uterus must be performed with great care if laceration of the fetus is to be avoided, particularly in cases of obstructed labour with a thin lower segment to which the fetal head is closely applied. Using the scalpel in the midline a horizontal 2-cm incision is made with very light pressure, such that only a few fibres are incised. Sweep the other index finger across this initial incision so that the layers can be seen with precision. Often only two or three very gentle strokes are required to go through the full thickness of the thin lower segment muscle. When partially through the muscle, press and release the centre of the incision with the forefinger: this should raise a 'bleb' of the very thin final layer so that it can be incised without risk to the underlying fetus. Alternatively, use the forefinger to stretch the incision and separate the few remaining muscle fibres to gain entry with blunt dissection. Once the uterus is entered, the forefinger is placed between the fetus and the uterine muscle towards one side and the incision is continued with either curved Mayo or bandage scissors. The same is repeated on the other side. After the initial entry incision, the lateral extensions should be directed upwards so that the final incision is a 'smile' of the 'Cheshire-cat' variety. About 80% of the incision is made with the scissors and then each forefinger is hooked into the angles, so the final extension of the incision is carried out with a pull of each forefinger. In cases in which the width of the lower segment is marginal, the angles of the incision may be directed almost vertically producing an enlarged 'trap-door' effect.

- If the fetus is in cephalic presentation, manual delivery of the head will usually be adequate. This entails inserting the flat of the lower hand without the thumb between the lower part of the incision and the fetal head. If the head is deeply engaged in the pelvis it may take considerable effort to elevate it up into the incision. It is important not to use a 'shoehorn' motion to achieve this as you risk extension of the uterine incision down into the vagina. Using the upper hand to grasp the wrist of the lower hand will often aid in elevation and reduce the amount of shoehorn motion. Once the head is elevated into the uterine incision it is flexed to produce the smallest diameter, following which sustained fundal pressure by the assistant should deliver the head through the uterine and abdominal wall incisions. If there is difficulty, and in some cases where the head is free and floating, forceps or the vacuum can be used to assist delivery of the head.
- In the case of breech presentation, the uterine incision is made in the same manner. As outlined in Chapter 8, the manoeuvres required for safe delivery of the breech are the same whether by the vaginal route or through a uterine incision. For all cases of breech delivery by caesarean

section, and particularly for those less than 36 weeks of gestation, the anaesthetist should have intravenous glyceryl trinitrate drawn up and ready to administer should head entrapment occur. This is a very real risk with the small breech, the body of which delivers easily through the lower segment while the larger after-coming head may become trapped, particularly with regional anaesthesia when there is no additional uterine relaxation (Robertson *et al.*1996). It is for these cases that the judicious administration of intravenous glyceryl trinitrate can assist atraumatic delivery of the fetal head (see Chapter 9).

- For the fetus in transverse lie delivery through a lower segment incision may, in some cases, be safely undertaken if the membranes are intact and the fetus can be turned to cephalic or breech presentation. Here again, intravenous glyceryl trinitrate may help to achieve this. If successful version has been performed, one has to decide whether the lower segment is sufficiently developed to allow this type of caesarean section or whether one has to move to the classical incision.
- Once the head of the infant is safely delivered, the anaesthetist should give five units of oxytocin intravenously, followed by an oxytocin infusion. Once separated, the placenta is delivered by controlled cord traction. After the placenta is delivered, the uterine cavity should be explored for remnants of placenta or membranes. This can be aided by use of a moistened gauze sponge over the hand.

It is inappropriate to routinely perform manual removal of the placenta. This is associated with greater blood loss, potential for infection and even occasional uterine inversion (Lasley et al. 1997). Unless the placenta is retained, manual removal at the time of caesarean section has no advantages (Wilkinson and Enkin 2000a).

Similarly, there is no reason to routinely bring the uterus out of the abdominal incision after delivery of the fetus and placenta (Wilkinson and Enkin 2000b). This can cause pain, nausea and vomiting in women under regional anaesthesia. Even for those with basic surgical skills there is adequate exposure to repair the uterine incision without this manoeuvre. On the other hand, if there is extension of the uterine incision or heavy bleeding that limits exposure, one should not hesitate to exteriorise the uterus. The ovaries and tubes can be checked without delivering the uterus through the incision.

Before closing the uterine incision Green-Armytage or ring forceps can be used to compress bleeding sinuses in the muscle edges. Even if there are no bleeders it is useful to place one forcep to identify the lower edge of the uterine incision. On occasions, the lower edge may be obscured by blood and the posterior wall of the uterine segment buckle forward and mimic, to the unwary, the lower edge of the uterine incision.

- Traditionally, closure of the uterine incision has been in two layers. A number of obstetricians have moved to single-layer closure. However, all of the previous literature on labour after caesarean section is based on two-layer closure. There are inadequate, and so far conflicting, data to say whether single-layer closure will have a greater, lesser or similar degree of scar integrity in a subsequent labour (Tucker *et al.* 1993; Chapman *et al.* 1997; Bujold *et al.* 2001). This question is being investigated in the CAESAR trial of single versus double layer closure. Until this trial is complete the authors recommend two-layer closure.

  The first layer is closed with a running or locking suture including the full thickness of uterine muscle. It is not necessary or desirable to include the decidua in this closure. After the first layer is inserted, pressure with a pack across the incision with one hand and uterine massage of the fundus with the other will compress the incision line and reduce bleeding. In single-layer closure no more sutures are added other than figure-of-eights if required for haemostasis.

  In double-layer closure it is best to make the first layer a running stitch as this avoids the bunched-up layering of a locking suture and facilitates the second level of sutures. It is common for the upper uterine edge of the incision to be much thicker than the lower. Hence, the second layer of sutures should raise a fold of muscle on the lower side, about 1 cm from the incision and the same on the upper side, including any unstitched muscle edge. In this manner the first layer of sutures is covered. The second layer can be running or locking, depending on haemostasis. In cases where there is sufficient upper and lower muscle thickness, such as primary elective section, the inner two-thirds can be stitched as the first layer followed by the outer third as the second layer. The assistant should keep good tension on the suture but not so much as to strangle or cut through the muscle.

  Most commonly 0 or No. 1 USP chromic or the polyglactin (Vicryl®, Ethicon) and polyglycolic acid (Dexon®, Davis & Geck)) sutures are used for the uterine incision, with the latter suture materials being preferable.

- There has been a trend not to close the uterovesical peritoneum and there are some data to support this (Nagele *et al.* 1996; Wilkinson and Enkin 2000c). However, not uncommonly, the peritoneal edge and underlying areolar tissue ooze and in such cases it is wise to close this layer with a running suture.

  For closure of the abdominal wall there is now evidence that the parietal peritoneum need not be closed (Luzuy *et al.* 1996). It is reasonable to loosely approximate the medial edges of the rectus muscles with two or three interrupted and lightly tied sutures. The rectus sheath is closed with a running suture and it is helpful to lock every third or fourth stitch. No sutures need be placed in the fat tissue – the less foreign material in the wound the less potential for infection. Indeed, all caesarean sections are at least potentially contaminated with the rich bacterial vaginal flora. The advantage of interrupted skin sutures is that serum can ooze out and is not sealed under the skin incision as a bacterial culture medium. If there is infection, one or two sutures can be removed to allow drainage, whereas with subcuticular sutures the entire area is sealed and drainage impossible. The long-term cosmetic effect of subcuticular versus interrupted wound skin staples or stitches is the same.

CLASSICAL CAESAREAN SECTION

The entry into the peritoneal cavity is as for the lower segment operation. With retraction, the vertical incision in the upper uterine segment can be made through a Pfannenstiel incision. The uterine incision is made with the scalpel starting in the upper part of the lower segment where the uterine wall is thin. Upon entry into the uterus the rest of the incision is extended upwards by 10–12 cm with scalpel and scissors, while the fingers protect the fetal parts. The lower limit of the incision is at the uterovesical peritoneal reflection. If the placenta is encountered under the incision, pass the hand to the nearest placental edge and, if necessary, enlarge the incision to deliver the fetus. Once the fetus and placenta are delivered it is usual to exteriorise the uterus for closure of the vertical incision. This is a much more vascular incision and it is helpful to have access to the uterus so that the assistant's hands can encircle the incision with the fingers on one side and the thumb on the other to compress the incision assisting its closure and reducing blood loss.

The uterine incision is closed in two or three layers. The first one or two layers, depending on the thickness of the muscle, are closed with a running suture to bring the deeper layers of uterine muscle together. When the deeper layers have been closed, such that the depth of incised uterine muscle not closed is about 1 cm, the final seromuscular layer is placed. This involves suturing approximately 1 cm from the edge of the incision with a continuous locking suture. The role of the assistant is important in compressing the line of the incision, both to reduce blood loss and take the pull off the sutures as they are placed so they do not cut through the muscle and allow the locking suture to be applied without undue tension.

LOW VERTICAL CAESAREAN SECTION

This requires more dissection of the bladder from the lower uterine segment to accommodate the vertical incision. Beware of dissecting off the bladder too much in the lateral aspects or you will excite much bleeding.

The initial vertical entry incision should be made with the same cautionary principles as the lower transverse incision. With a finger protecting the fetal presenting part, the incision is extended up and down with scissors. The main problem is a balance between extending too far downwards into the vascular vagina and too far up into the upper uterine segment. Once the incision is made the lower end can be stitched and held as a stay suture. This helps to prevent extension of the incision into the bladder and vagina, as well as delineating the lower edge to facilitate closure of the uterine wound.

The principles of closure of the uterine incision are the same as for the transverse incision.

Finally, a surgical report should be written, including the indications for and a description of the operation. In particular, details of extensions of the uterine incision or encroachment into the upper uterine segment will help those involved in a subsequent pregnancy to make reasoned decisions about the next delivery. During the postoperative hospital stay, a review of the above factors should also be held with the patient.

To reduce the risks of atelectasis and thromboembolism, postoperative care should emphasise deep breathing and chest physiotherapy as well as leg exercises and early ambulation.

References

Bethune M, Permezel M. (1997) The relationship between gestational age and the incidence of classical caesarean section. *Aust N Z J Obstet Gynaecol* 37:153–5.

Boyle JG, Gabbe SG. (1996) T and J vertical extensions in low transverse cesarean births. *Obstet Gynecol* 87:238–43.

Bujold E, Bujold C, Gauthier RJ. (2001) Uterine rupture during a trial of labor after one-versus two-layer closure of a low transverse cesarean. [Abstract.] *Am J Obstet Gynecol* 184:S18.

Chapman SJ, Owen J, Hauth JC. (1997) One-versus two-layer closure of a low transverse cesarean: the next pregnancy. *Am J Obstet Gynecol* 89:16–18.

Darj E, Nordstrom ML. (1999) Misgav Ladach method for cesarean section compared to Pfannenstiel method. *Acta Obstet Gynecol Scand* 78:37–41.

Drife J, Walker J, editors. (2001) Caesarean section: current practice. *Clin Obstet Gynaecol* 15:1–194.

Guihard P, Blondel B. (2001) Trends in risk factors for caesarean sections in France between 1981 and 1995: lessons for reducing the rates in the future. *Br J Obstet Gynaecol* 108:48–55.

Hannah ME, Hannah WJ, Hewson SA, Hodnett ED, Saigal S, Willam AR. (2002) Planned caesarean section versus planned vaginal birth for breech presentation at term: a randomised multicentre trial. *Lancet* 356:1375–83.

Hopkins L, Smaill F. (2000) Antibiotic prophylaxis regimens and drugs for caesarean section. *Cochrane Database Syst Rev* (2).

Lasley DS, Eblen A, Yancey MK, Duff P. (1997) The effects of placental removal method on the incidence of post-cesarean infections. *Am J Obstet Gynecol* 176:1250–4.

Luzuy F, Irion O, Beguin F. (1996) Non-closure of the visceral and parietal layers of the peritoneum at caesarean section: a randomised controlled trial. *Br J Obstet Gynaecol* 103:690–4.

Nagele F, Karas H, Spitzer D, Staudach A. (1996) Closure or non-closure of the visceral peritoneum at cesarean delivery. *Am J Obstet Gynecol* 174:1366–70.

Paterson-Brown S, Amu O. (1998) Should doctors perform an elective caesarean section on request? *BMJ* 317:462–5.

RCOG. (1995) Report of the RCOG Working Party On Prophylaxis Against Thromboembolism In Gynaecology And Obstetrics. London: Royal College of Obstetricians and Gynaecologists.

Robertson PA, Foran CM, Croughan-Minichane MS, Kilpatrick SJ. (1996) Head entrapment and neonatal outcome by mode of delivery in breech deliveries from 28 to 36 weeks of gestation. *Am J Obstet Gynecol* 174:1742–9.

Savage W. (2000) The caesarean section epidemic. *J Obstet Gynaecol* 20:223–5.

Stark M, Finkel A. (1994) Comparison between the Joel Cohen and Pfannenstiel incisions in caesarean section. *Eur J Obstet Gynecol Reprod Biol* 53:121–2.

Tucker JM, Hauth JC, Hodgkins P. (1993) Trial of labor after one-or two-layer closure of a low transverse uterine incision. *Am J Obstet Gynecol* 168:545–6.

Tully L, Gates S, Brocklehurst P, McHarg K McK, Ayers S. (2002) Surgical techniques used during caesarean section operations: results of a national survey of practice in the UK. *Eur J Obstet Gynecol Reprod Biol* 102:120–6.

Wilkinson C, Enkin MW. (2000a) Manual removal of the placenta at caesarean section. *Cochrane Database Syst Rev* (2).

Wilkinson C, Enkin MW. (2000b) Uterine exteriorisation versus intraperitoneal repair at caesarean section. *Cochrane Database Syst Rev* (2).

Wilkinson C, Enkin MW. (2000c) Peritoneal non-closure at caesarean section. *Cochrane Database Syst Rev* (2).

11 Vaginal birth after caesarean section

Over the last 20 years, caesarean section rates have risen worldwide. In many developed countries the overall caesarean section rates range between 15% and 25%, while approximately 10% of the obstetric population have been previously delivered by caesarean section. Thus, about one in ten pregnant women, and those looking after them, need to consider the implications for pregnancy, labour and delivery after previous caesarean section. The main consideration is the balance between the risks and benefits of repeat elective caesarean section versus trial for vaginal delivery.

Selection

The most dreaded complication is, of course, uterine rupture (Chapter 12). Thus, a trial for vaginal delivery can only be contemplated when the appropriate personnel and facilities are available. Anaesthesia, nursing, and obstetric staff should be immediately available, together with the appropriate operating facilities and blood transfusion. These have been reviewed in national guidelines (SOGC 1997; ACOG 1999).

The principle of informed consent is important. The woman should understand the maternal risks involved with caesarean section – both elective and after failed trial for vaginal delivery (Irvine and Shaw 1997). The possibility of complete uterine rupture in labour (approximately 3–5/1000) should be presented along with the rare risk of perinatal damage should rupture occur (Appleton *et al.* 2000; Smith *et al* 2002).

There are certain individual factors in the woman's past obstetric history that may help predict the likelihood of successful labour and vaginal delivery.

- Vaginal delivery before or after the previous caesarean section increases the likelihood of a successful trial and vaginal delivery in a subsequent pregnancy (Zelop *et al.*2000).
- The timing of the previous caesarean section in labour is an important guide to the type of uterine strain and work required in the next

pregnancy (Arulkumaran *et al.* 1989). Thus, the woman who had a previous caesarean section, either with no labour or in the latent phase of labour, will exhibit the stronger pattern of uterine work similar to that of the nulliparous woman, whereas the woman with a previous caesarean section in the active phase of labour (fully effaced cervix, greater than 3 cm dilatation) will show a multiparous pattern of labour with less uterine work.

- If the previous caesarean section was for dystocia, the chance of successful subsequent vaginal delivery is reduced but not enough to preclude a trial if other factors are favourable (ACOG 1999).
- Women who have had more than one previous lower transverse segment caesarean section may labour and deliver successfully but the risk of uterine rupture is increased and they should be aware of this (Leung *et al.* 1993; Bretelle *et al.* 2001).
- An interpregnancy interval of less than six months may be associated with a higher risk of uterine scar disruption (Esposito *et al.* 2000).
- The woman with twins in the next pregnancy is a controversial candidate for trial of vaginal delivery. Overdistension of the uterus with twins and the possibility of intrauterine manipulation for delivery of the second twin increases the potential risk of rupture in this group, although success has been reported (Miller *et al.* 1996).
- Preliminary studies suggest that ultrasonographic measurement of the lower uterine segment may help to select those with a higher risk of scar rupture (Rozenburg *et al.* 1999; Gotoh *et al.* 2000). Further work is needed to delineate the clinical role of this promising approach.

Thus, a consideration of the blend of above factors should allow the woman and her doctor to make a reasonably informed decision.

Contraindications

The following factors militate against labour after previous caesarean section:

- Any uterine scar that encroaches on the upper uterine segment is a contraindication to subsequent labour. These include previous classical caesarean section, hysterotomy and many cases of low vertical caesarean section. In spite of the name of the latter, the incision often encroaches into the upper uterine segment. Marked extension of a transverse lower segment caesarean section incision, and particularly the 'inverted T' type, are best not subjected to labour.

- Myomectomy incisions that have involved full thickness of the uterine wall and entry into the cavity are probably more vulnerable to rupture than partial thickness incisions.
- Previous uterine rupture.
- Other obstetric complications that contraindicate labour, such as placenta praevia and transverse lie.
- Individual factors such as maternal age, secondary infertility, previous perinatal loss, etc, may obviously influence the decision against labour.

The women must be informed and committed. Coercion, subtle or otherwise, is inappropriate.

Management

ANTENATAL CARE

Apart from the detailed review of the factors noted above, antenatal care should be routine.

There is no evidence that pelvimetry is of any value, although ultrasound estimates of fetal weight may be useful in making a decision regarding delivery in some cases.

INDUCTION OF LABOUR

Spontaneous labour is always preferable to induced labour and only women who are well-established for induction should be considered. Provided that there is a valid reason for induction and the cervix is favourable, amniotomy is the method of choice. This may be followed by the careful administration of intravenous oxytocin if progressive labour does not ensue.

There are a number of reviews, mainly from tertiary-level hospitals, that suggest the judicious use of oxytocin and prostaglandins for cervical ripening and induction of labour is reasonable in women with one previous transverse lower segment caesarean section. However, reports have shown a significantly increased risk of rupture with the use of prostaglandins (Wing *et al.* 1998; Ravasia *et al.* 2000; Lydon-Rochelle *et al.* 2001). This is particularly so with, but not limited to, misoprostol (Plaut *et al.* 1998; Wing *et al.* 1998). If the cervix is unfavourable, the use of prostaglandins should be approached with extreme caution and the woman informed that their use increases the risk of rupture.

LABOUR

The woman with a previous caesarean section should be advised to come into hospital early in labour. In the early stages, if all is normal, it is reasonable to allow her to ambulate. Once labour is established it is prudent to insert an intravenous drip. Blood should be taken for group and screen.

Epidural analgesia may be provided as indicated for any other labour. The theoretical worry that epidural would mask the pain and tenderness of uterine rupture has not been substantiated.

Continuous electronic fetal heart rate monitoring is not routinely indicated early in the labour. However, when labour becomes active it is beneficial as one of the earliest signs of uterine dehiscence is abnormality of the fetal heart rate.

The progress of labour should be carefully charted using a partogram. To be safe, one should expect a smooth and progressive labour. Although one tries to manage the labour in as normal a manner as possible, this is not a normal labour and the risks to the mother and infant are increased. Discretion is usually the better part of valour if labour is non-progressive. Oxytocin augmentation of non-progressive labour should only be considered in hospitals with on-site obstetric and anaesthetic personnel. If augmentation is undertaken, one should anticipate a smooth progressive response and if this does not occur a repeat caesarean section should be performed.

While there are a number of reassuring studies about the use of oxytocics to induce and augment labour, these are not large enough to provide complete security. Furthermore, the fact remains that oxytocic use is commonly implicated in most large reviews of uterine rupture after previous caesarean section (Baskett and Kieser 2001; ACOG 2002). Thus, the administration of oxytocics should only be considered with careful thought and after informing the woman that this increases the risk to her and the infant, albeit by a small amount. These points have been emphasised in the fifth report of the Confidential Enquiry into Stillbirths and Deaths in Infancy (1998).

A careful watch is kept for signs and symptoms of early uterine rupture. These are by no means consistent but can include:

- persistent pain and tenderness over the lower uterine segment between uterine contractions – this can be hard to interpret as a minor degree of these symptoms may exist in normal labour
- in the thin woman, central or unilateral swelling over the lower uterine segment may be detected
- maternal hypotension, tachycardia and syncope
- vaginal bleeding

- the bladder is often adherent to the site of a lower segment caesarean scar and, therefore, haematuria may be one of the early signs if the integrity of the scar and adherent bladder wall is disrupted
- fetal heart rate abnormality is the most consistent and reliable early warning sign; this may include tachycardia, late and variable decelerations – with persistent bradycardia the most worrying.

The picture of catastrophic uterine rupture with sudden severe lower abdominal pain, cessation of uterine contractions, vaginal bleeding, dramatic elevation of the presenting part, fetal death and signs of intra-abdominal haemorrhage is rare with previous low transverse caesarean scar rupture. The transverse lower segment scar is thin, relatively avascular and may dehisce with minimal clinical signs.

There is now considerable published evidence to support vaginal delivery after previous caesarean section in selected women. In many hospitals, up to 50% of the women who previously delivered by caesarean section may expect to safely deliver vaginally in a subsequent pregnancy. However, no large randomised trial has compared trial of vaginal delivery with elective repeat caesarean section. A meta-analysis of studies from the 1990s suggests a slightly increased risk of the rare events of uterine rupture and neonatal morbidity and mortality with a trial for vaginal delivery and an increased rate of maternal morbidity with elective caesarean section (Mozurkewich and Hutton 2000).

As with many areas of medicine the problem is the 'pendulum syndrome', when excessive zeal in attempts to achieve vaginal delivery leads to unreasonable risk. With careful selection, the majority of women will have a smooth and progressive labour, achieving vaginal delivery with minimal risk to themselves and the infant. When additional risk factors and interventions are added, the risk of scar rupture increases with very little gain in the number of vaginal deliveries achieved. This is yet another area of obstetrics where sensible clinical balance is required.

References

ACOG. (1999) *Vaginal Birth after Previous Cesarean Delivery. Practice Bulletin No. 5.* Washington DC: American College of Obstetricians and Gynecologists.

ACOG. (2002) *Induction of labor for vaginal birth after cesarean delivery. Committee Opinion No. 271.* Washington DC: American College of Obstetricians and Gynecologists.

Appleton B, Targett C, Rasumssen M, VBAC Study Group. (2000) Vaginal birth after caesarean section: an Australian multicentre study. *Aust N Z J Obstet Gynaecol* 40:87–91.

Arulkumaran S, Gibb DMF, Ingemarsson I, Kitchener HS, Ratnam SS. (1989) Uterine activity during spontaneous labour after previous lower-segment caesarean section. *Br J Obstet Gynaecol* 96:933–8.

Baskett TF, Kieser KE. (2001) A 10-year population-based study of uterine rupture. [Abstract.] *Obstet Gynecol* 2001;97:S69.

Bretelle F, Cravello L, Shojai R, D'ercole RV, Blanc B. (2001) Vaginal birth after two previous cesarean sections. *Eur J Obstet Gynecol Reprod Biol* 94:23–6.

Confidential Enquiry into Stillbirths and Deaths in Infancy. (1998) *5th Annual Report*. London: Maternal and Child Health Research Consortium.

Esposito MA, Menihan CA, Malee MP. (2000) Association of interpregnancy interval with uterine scar failure in labor: a case-control study. *Am J Obstet Gynecol* 183:1180–3.

Gotoh H, Masuzaki H, Yoshida A, Yoshimura S, Miyamura T, Ishimaru J. (2000) Predicting incomplete uterine rupture with vaginal sonography during the late second trimester in women with prior cesarean. *Obstet Gynecol* 95:596–600.

Irvine LM, Shaw RW. (2001) Trial of scar or elective repeat caesarean section at maternal request? *J Obstet Gynaecol* 21:463–7.

Leung AS, Farmer RM, Leung EK, Mediaris AL, Paul RH. (1993) Risk factors associated with uterine rupture during trial of labor after cesarean delivery: a case-control study. *Am J Obstet Gynecol* 168:1358–63.

Lydon-Rochelle M, Holt VL, Easterling TR, Martin DP. (2001) Risk of uterine rupture among women with a prior cesarean delivery. *N Engl J Med* 345:3–8.

Miller DA, Mullin P, Hou D, Paul RH. (1996) Vaginal birth after cesarean section in twin gestation. *Am J Obstet Gynecol* 175:194–8.

Mozurkewich EL, Hutton EK. (2000) Elective repeat cesarean delivery versus trial of labor: a meta-analysis of the literature from 1989 to 1999. *Am J Obstet Gynecol* 183:1187–97.

Plaut MM, Schwartz ML, Lubarsky SL. (1998) Uterine rupture associated with the use of misoprostol in the gravid patient with a previous cesarean section. *Am J Obstet Gynecol* 180:1535–42.

Ravasia DJ, Wood SL, Pollard JK. (2000) Uterine rupture during induced trial of labor among women with previous cesarean delivery. *Am J Obstet Gynecol* 183:1176–9.

Rozenberg P, Goffinet F, Philippe HJ, Nisand I. (1999) Thickness of the lower segment: its influence in the management of patients with previous cesarean sections. *Eur J Obstet Gynecol Reprod Biol* 87:39–45.

Smith GCS, Pell JP, Cameron AD, Dobbie R. (2002) Risk of perinatal death associated with labour after previous cesarean delivery in uncomplicated term pregnancies. *JAMA* 287: 2684–90.

SOGC (Society of Obstetricians and Gynaecologists of Canada). (1997) Clinical Practice Guidelines. Vaginal birth after previous caesarean birth. *J Soc Obstet Gynaecol Can* 19:1425–8.

Wing DA, Lovett K, Paul RH. (1998) Disruption of prior uterine incision following misoprostol for labor induction in women with previous cesarean delivery. *Obstet Gynecol* 1998;91:828–30.

Zelop CM, Shipp TD, Repke JT, Cohen A, Lieberman E. (2000) Effect of previous vaginal delivery on the risk of uterine rupture during a subsequent trial of labour. *Am J Obstet Gynecol* 183:1184–6.

12 Uterine rupture and emergency obstetric hysterectomy

The hospital incidence of uterine rupture varies from one in100–500 deliveries in developing countries to one in 5000–6000 with well-developed hospital services.

The type of rupture may be complete, involving the full thickness of the uterine wall, with or without extrusion of fetal parts, or incomplete, when the uterine muscle has separated but the visceral peritoneum remains intact. Other than separation of previous uterine scars, the most common site of complete rupture is the anterior lower uterine segment. Rupture may be more prominent laterally and involve bleeding into the broad ligament and retroperitoneal space. Less common is rupture of both the distended lower segment and the vaginal fornix. In 5–10% of cases the rupture involves the bladder wall.

Causes

UTERINE SCAR

Rupture of a previous caesarean section scar is by far the most common cause in developed countries. Scars that encroach upon the upper uterine segment are more prone to rupture because this contractile part of the uterus may disrupt healing of the scar during the puerperium. Estimates of uterine rupture associated with pregnancy and labour vary:

- classical incision 4–9%
- low vertical incision 1–7%
- low transverse incision 0.2–1.5% (details of this cause of uterine rupture are covered in Chapter 11).

Although there is less documented experience, hysterotomy incisions seem to behave in the same manner as those of classical caesarean section.

Myomectomy scars that are not large and do not involve the full thickness of the uterine wall are not prone to rupture. However, those that are extensive, and particularly if they involve full thickness of the uterine wall, are more likely to rupture.

Other events that may scar and weaken the uterine wall to a greater or lesser degree include uteroplasty, salpingectomy with deep cornual resection, previous uterine perforation, repeated and excessive curettage and operative hysteroscopy. Deep cervical scars associated with conisation, amputation and cerclage may risk rupture if they encroach on the lower uterine segment.

OBSTRUCTED LABOUR

This is the most common cause in developing countries and the main predisposing factors are cephalopelvic disproportion, malpresentations, such as transverse lie, and fetal anomaly, such as hydrocephalus. The multiparous uterus is most vulnerable as it often responds to obstruction with stronger uterine contractions, whereas the nulliparous uterus will tend to react with diminished uterine activity. In this context, oxytocin augmentation of non-progressive labour in the multiparous patient should only be undertaken with considerable caution.

TRAUMA

Obstetric uterine trauma should be extremely rare in well-run maternity services but may be caused by internal version and breech extraction, forceps rotation, fetal destructive operations, shoulder dystocia and manual removal of an accretic placenta.

- Traumatic laceration of the uterus can occur in association with surgical termination of pregnancy in the first 20 weeks of gestation.
- External trauma, such as a motor vehicle accident, is a relatively rare cause.

MISCELLANEOUS

There are a number of rare specific conditions that can predispose to uterine rupture, such as:

- uterine anomalies
- gestational trophoblastic disease
- placenta accreta, increta and percreta
- cornual pregnancy,
- severe concealed placental abruption.

In general, the multiparous uterus is much more vulnerable to uterine rupture as repeated pregnancy leads to fibrosis and thinning of the uterine muscle.

The clinical features of uterine rupture may vary from an obvious intra-abdominal haemorrhagic catastrophe to very mild and non-specific signs, as outlined in Chapter 11.

Management

Treat hypovolaemia with intravenous crystalloid and blood products as necessary.

Perform laparotomy and remove the fetus and placenta. It is essential to rapidly secure haemostasis. To achieve this the uterus is brought up out of the incision. The assistant's hands are placed behind the uterus and, with the thumbs and index fingers at each side, the uterine vessels can be occluded. The extent of the uterine rupture can then be delineated and the bleeding edges occluded with Green-Armytage or ring forceps. If uterine conservation is desirable, bilateral uterine and ovarian artery ligation may be swiftly performed (see Chapter 16). If the uterine laceration is simple and the desire for future reproduction strong, it may be acceptable just to repair the laceration, provided haemostasis is secured. Alternatively, repair of the rupture and tubal ligation may be appropriate. In all cases, the procedures should be covered by perioperative antibiotics and the integrity of the bladder wall should always be checked.

Many patients with uterine rupture will require hysterectomy and this is considered below.

Emergency obstetric hysterectomy

The indications for and mortality associated with emergency obstetric hysterectomy vary with the type of obstetric services available. The three main conditions leading to emergency obstetric hysterectomy are placenta accreta and/or praevia, uterine rupture and uterine atony. Mortality ranges from 0–25%, depending on the level of hospital care. Maternal morbidity is common due to haemorrhage, disseminated intravascular coagulation, blood transfusion, infection and potential urological injury to the bladder and ureter.

SURGICAL ASPECTS

- Major vessel ligation of the uterine, ovarian or internal iliac arteries can be used to try and rapidly reduce haemorrhage and, in selected cases, may allow preservation of the uterus (see Chapter 16).

- Subtotal hysterectomy maybe chosen if the cervix and paracolpos are not involved in the rupture or haemorrhagic site. This is simpler, faster and less likely to injure the lower urinary tract than total hysterectomy. In many cases of uterine rupture, subtotal hysterectomy is a good example of surgical discretion being the better part of valour.
- Total hysterectomy is required if the cervix or paracolpos are involved in the uterine laceration, or if there is marked sepsis.
- Many of the pedicles are very thick, oedematous and vascular. Therefore, they should be doubly clamped and ligated. To avoid haematoma formation, place a free tie proximally and a second transfixing suture distal to the free tie.
- Pedicles are more likely to remain secure if they are smaller, placed in the correct anatomical plane (avoid twisting) and have a generous tissue pedicle distal to the ligature.
- To avoid the ureter, after clamping the uterine arteries place all other clamps medially.
- In many cases of uterine rupture, the integrity of the bladder wall is vulnerable. This is particularly so in cases of ruptured lower segment scars to which the bladder is often adherent. In most cases, therefore, it is appropriate to test the integrity of the bladder wall intraoperatively with dye or sterile milk inserted through the Foley catheter.
- When performing a total hysterectomy it can be quite difficult to identify the cervix. This may be helped by placing a finger down through the uterine incision into the vagina and hooking it up to identify the rim of the cervix. The vagina should then be entered posteriorly and the incision carefully guided laterally and anteriorly.
- Perioperative antibiotics should be continued for at least 48 hours.
- Institute postoperative thromboprophylaxis.

After such a potentially catastrophic event detailed perioperative notes should be placed in the chart. A debriefing session of all involved staff is advisable. The patient and her partner should be counselled by an experienced obstetrician.

Further reading

Aboyeji AP, Ijaiya MDA, Yahaya UR. (2001) Ruptured uterus: a study of 100 consecutive cases in Ilorin, Nigeria. *J Obstet Gynaecol Res* 27:341–8.

Al-Sakka M, Hamsho A, Khan L. (1998) Rupture of the pregnant uterus: a 21 year review. *Int J Gynaecol Obstet* 63:105–8.

Gardeil F, Daley S, Turner MJ. (1994) Uterine rupture in pregnancy reviewed. *Eur J Obstet Gynecol Reprod Biol* 56:107–110.

Miller DA, Goodwin TM, Gherman RV, Paul RH. (1997) Intrapartum rupture of the unscarred uterus. *Obstet Gynecol* 89:671–3.

Soltan MH, Khashoggi T, Adelusi B. (1996) Pregnancy following rupture of the pregnant uterus. *Int J Gynaecol Obstet* 52:37–42.

Turner MJ. (2002) Uterine rupture. *Clin Obstet Gynaecol* 16:69–80.

Zelop CM, Harlow BL, Frigoletto FD. (1993) Emergency peripartum hysterectomy. *Am J Obstet Gynecol* 168:1443–8.

13 Shoulder dystocia

Shoulder dystocia occurs when there is failure of the shoulders to deliver spontaneously or with gentle downward traction on the fetal head. It is diagnosed when the head is delivered but external rotation does not occur, the head recedes with the chin firmly against the vulva and the neck is not visible or palpable. The diagnosis is, to some extent, in the eye of the beholder and this accounts for the relatively wide range of incidence: 0.2–2.0% of cephalic vaginal deliveries. It has been suggested that a more standard definition may be a head-to-completion-of-delivery interval greater than 60 seconds or the use of ancillary manoeuvres to effect delivery of the shoulders (Spong *et al.* 1995). However, even in normal deliveries without shoulder dystocia, the head may deliver with the final push of one contraction and the shoulders and rest of the infant after awaiting the next contraction. The potential for damage to the infant from asphyxia and trauma is such that this condition has assumed considerable clinical and medico-legal significance (Leigh and James 1998).

Mechanism

The anteroposterior diameter of the pelvic brim is narrower than the oblique and transverse diameters. The bisacromial diameter of the term fetus is larger than the biparietal diameter. It is, therefore, the flexibility of the shoulders that allows their rotation, accommodation and descent through the pelvis. In spontaneous delivery, as the head passes through the pelvic outlet, the posterior fetal shoulder descends through the sciatic notch or the sacral bay, while the anterior shoulder is accommodated in the retropubic space. If the bisacromial diameter is large and the shoulders attempt to enter the pelvic brim via the narrow anteroposterior diameter shoulder dystocia may occur. In general, the posterior shoulder will descend below the sacral promontory and it is the anterior shoulder that becomes impacted above and behind the pubic symphysis. On rare occasions, both anterior and posterior shoulders may arrest above the pelvic brim – bilateral shoulder dystocia. This requires considerable extension of the head and neck and is usually associated with assisted mid-pelvic delivery.

When the head has delivered, the supply of oxygen to the fetus is reduced for two reasons:

- the uterus contracts down, which reduces or stops the blood flow to the intervillous space
- the fetal chest is compressed so that, even though the infant's mouth and nose are delivered, effective respiratory effort is not possible.

It has been shown that, after delivery of the fetal head, the progression of hypoxia is such that the umbilical artery pH falls at a rate of 0.04 units per minute (Wood *et al.* 1973).

Fetal complications

ASPHYXIA

For the reasons cited above, the fetus is subjected to increasing hypoxia after delivery of the head. Provided that the oxygen supply was normal up until delivery of the head there should be four to six minutes before the likelihood of permanent hypoxic damage. However, if there was an element of hypoxia before delivery of the head, serious asphyxia may occur in a shorter time. In addition, a combination of hypoxia, trauma and obstructed cerebral venous return may combine to further damage the fetal brain (CESDI 1998).

BRACHIAL PLEXUS INJURY

This is one of the most dreaded neonatal complications and has increasing medico-legal connotations. Some 5–15% of neonates born after shoulder dystocia will suffer brachial plexus palsy of the Erb–Duchenne type involving nerve roots C5 and C6. Only rarely is there injury to the whole brachial plexus, leading to a flail arm. The least common injury is Klumpke's palsy, caused by damage to the nerves roots C8 and T1. The risk of permanent injury is usually in the 5–30% range. Most reports show less than 10% long-term disability, although two reviews found a more pessimistic long-term outcome, with failed resolution of the palsy in up to 50% of cases (Eng *et al.* 1996; Bager 1997).

FRACTURE

The clavicle is the most likely to fracture and this occurs in about 15% of infants with shoulder dystocia. Fracture of the humerus does occur but much less commonly (less than 1%). On rare occasions, potentially disastrous fractures of the cervical spine can occur in association with twisting manoeuvres of the fetal head.

It is emphasised that fractures of the clavicle and humerus, when recognised and treated, heal well with no long-term sequelae. While they may be distressing to the attendant, the patient and observers, they are acknowledged complications of the condition and the manoeuvres required to treat it and do not have the same long-term implications as brachial plexus injury or severe and sustained hypoxia.

Maternal complications

GENITAL TRACT LACERATIONS

There is often extension of the episiotomy or other lacerations of the lower genital tract because of the additional vaginal manoeuvres. Uterine rupture may occur on rare occasions in association with vigorous uterine manipulation.

POSTPARTUM HAEMORRHAGE

This is more common because of bleeding from lacerations and uterine atony.

Predisposing factors

ANTEPARTUM

The following factors, many of which are interrelated, increase the risk of shoulder dystocia (Baskett 2001):

- fetal macrosomia is by far the most common cause and often a factor in other predisposing conditions
- maternal diabetes: infants of diabetic mothers have a greater shoulder/head circumference ratio due to the insulin sensitive nature of the tissues that make up shoulder girth. Such infants have a higher risk of shoulder dystocia compared with non-diabetic infants of similar weight
- maternal obesity
- excessive maternal weight gain in pregnancy
- post-term pregnancy: due to the higher incidence of macrosomia with prolonged pregnancy. The fetal chest and shoulders will continue to grow steadily post-term, whereas the biparietal diameter growth tends to plateau, increasing the shoulder/head circumference ratio
- previous shoulder dystocia.

INTRAPARTUM

Although the majority of cases with shoulder dystocia show normal progression in labour leading to spontaneous or low pelvis assisted delivery, there are certain patterns of labour that increase the likelihood of shoulder dystocia:

- protracted or arrested active phase of the late first stage of labour
- protracted or arrested descent in the second stage of labour
- assisted mid pelvis delivery.

Prediction and prevention

Efforts have been made to find accurate predictive factors so that a prevention strategy for shoulder dystocia and its sequelae could be found. Unfortunately, these have been unsuccessful. The main problem is that the predisposing factors are common and the condition they aim to predict, shoulder dystocia, is not. Furthermore, injury associated with shoulder dystocia is even less common. The main risk factor is macrosomia and the ability to predict this is unreliable. The hope that ultrasound would give a more precise prediction of macrosomia has not been substantiated, particularly at higher fetal weights where clinical estimate has been shown to be as accurate (Delpapa and Mueller-Heubach 1991; Chauhan *et al.* 1998; Sherman *et al.* 1998). Attempts to refine the ultrasound measurements using shoulder width as a predictor for shoulder dystocia have also been unsuccessful (Verspyck *et al.* 1999). Macrosomia is undoubtedly the most important predisposing factor to shoulder dystocia and yet the majority of cases occur in infants weighing less than 4500 g. It has been suggested that if the fetal weight was predicted to be greater than 4500 g, elective caesarean section would be justified. However, the futility of such a policy was demonstrated by a decision–analysis model which showed that, for each permanent brachial plexus injury prevented by elective caesarean section for estimated fetal weight greater than 4500 g, 3695 caesarean sections would have to be performed (Rouse *et al.* 1996). The additional cost to the health service in the USA would be $8.7million. A review of obstetric brachial palsy shows that just over 50% of all cases involve shoulder dystocia (Pollack *et al.* 2000). However, there is reasonable evidence from electromyographic studies that some cases of brachial plexus palsy originate *in utero*. There are also observational studies that the palsy may be due to the shoulder dystocia itself rather than the manoeuvres used to overcome it. Excessive downward traction on the head to overcome shoulder dystocia has always been incriminated as the main cause of the brachial plexus palsy.

However, a number of studies show that in up to one-third of cases it is the posterior shoulder in which the palsy occurs, suggesting that impaction of the posterior shoulder at the sacral promontory may be the cause (Walle and Hartikainen-Sorie 1993).

The recurrence rate of shoulder dystocia has been reviewed and shows a risk of recurrence from 1.1 to 16.7% (Smith *et al.* 1994; Baskett and Allen 1995; Flannelly and Simm 1995; Lewis *et al.* 1995; Olugbile and Mascarenhas 2000; Ginsberg and Moisidis 2001). The increased risk varied from two-fold to 16-fold. One study has reported a 33% recurrence risk with previous brachial plexus palsy – obviously a very high-risk group (Al-Quattam and Al-Kharfy 1996).

Unfortunately, therefore, we are left with predisposing factors that are common and lack clinically applicable predictive value. Furthermore, the majority of cases of shoulder dystocia occur without identifiable risk factors. Nonetheless, an awareness and appraisal of cumulative risk factors should lead to a cautious approach in selected cases. For example, the woman who had a previous shoulder dystocia without injury is probably suitable for subsequent vaginal delivery provided that there are no additional risk factors and the patient is fully informed. On the contrary, the woman who had a previous shoulder dystocia and brachial plexus palsy, particularly if the injury was significant and sustained, is probably better delivered by elective caesarean section in a subsequent pregnancy. The woman with diabetes and a fetal weight estimated above 4250 g is probably more safely delivered by caesarean section. Certain patterns of labour, such as a protracted late first stage of labour, slow descent in the second stage and the need for assisted mid-pelvis delivery may, in the presence of clinically diagnosed macrosomia, dictate that delivery by caesarean section would be more prudent.

Management

The classic presentation is that the head delivers, either spontaneously or assisted, does not undergo external rotation and recoils tightly against the perineum – the so called 'turtle sign'. If there has been no concomitant hypoxia it is reasonable to await the next contraction and bearing-down effort for the shoulders to rotate and make their way through the pelvic brim. If this does not occur and gentle downward traction on the head fails to deliver the anterior shoulder then the presence of shoulder dystocia is clear. It is very important not to put strong downward force on the head against the unyielding anterior shoulder impacted behind the pubic symphysis – this is the most common cause of brachial plexus palsy associated with shoulder dystocia. As the problem lies at the level of the pelvic brim, traction or twisting of the fetal head and neck are illogical, potentially traumatic and will not work. Once shoulder dystocia is diagnosed, additional personnel should be summoned to assist in providing analgesia and neonatal resuscitation and to guide the woman into positions most favourable to assist delivery of the shoulders.

The situation should be decisively explained to the patient. Provide inhalation analgesia (if not under epidural analgesia), apply local anaesthesia to the perineum, if this not already in place, perform a generous episiotomy and proceed with the manoeuvres necessary to assist delivery of the shoulders.

MCROBERTS' MANOEUVRE

This manoeuvre is simple and the least traumatic to the fetus and mother. It will overcome the majority of mild to moderate cases of shoulder dystocia and is recommended as the first line of treatment (Gonik *et al.* 1983). The maternal hips are sharply flexed against her abdomen. The effect on the pelvic brim is to rotate the symphysis superiorly and straighten the lumbosacral angle. This helps to facilitate the descent of the posterior shoulder below the sacral promontory and, by flexing the fetal spine towards the anterior shoulder, may help to dislodge that shoulder. It also reduces the angle of inclination of the pelvis, bringing the plane of the pelvic inlet perpendicular to the expulsive forces required for delivery. A series of engineering studies have been applied to this manoeuvre showing that it does reduce the extraction forces necessary to deliver the shoulders (Gonik *et al.* 1989). In addition, the rate of application of force was found to be important, as fetal injury was greater when the same force was applied rapidly compared with slowly and uniformly (Allen *et al.* 1994).

ROTATE THE FETAL SHOULDERS TO THE OBLIQUE DIAMETER: DIRECTIONAL SUPRAPUBIC PRESSURE

As the anteroposterior diameter of the pelvic brim is the narrowest, it is logical to try to rotate the shoulders to the wider oblique and transverse diameters. This should not be attempted by twisting the neck. Usually one cannot insert fingers between the head and neck anteriorly and reach the anterior shoulder. It is best to insert two fingers posteriorly in the vagina and by pressure on the scapula push the infant's posterior shoulder off the midline to the oblique diameter. The posterior shoulder is usually accessible, as it has descended below the sacral promontory.

Directed suprapubic pressure may be used to assist disimpaction of the anterior shoulder and rotation to the oblique diameter. This is best applied with the heel of the hand behind the shoulder, downwards and lateral.

Rubin showed that the adducted diameter of the shoulders is narrower than the abducted diameter, making pressure on the back of the shoulder the most logical technique (Rubin 1964). There is advantage in rotating the fetal shoulders to the wider oblique diameter before or along with all other manoeuvres.

WOODS' SCREW MANOEUVRE

Almost 60 years ago, Woods studied the relationship between the shoulders and bony pelvis during delivery (Woods 1943). Using wooden models he showed that the relationship between the symphysis, sacral promontory and coccyx and the fetal shoulders was similar to the threads of a screw. He therefore demonstrated that trying to pull or push impacted fetal shoulders through the pelvis was illogical and traumatic. However, they could be 'corkscrewed' through the pelvis by rotating the shoulders 180 degrees. To achieve this, he placed two fingers on the anterior aspect of the accessible posterior shoulder in the sacral bay and exerted pressure to rotate the baby 180 degrees, thereby rotating the posterior shoulder, which started below the level of the pelvic brim, to the anterior position, making it accessible for delivery. This is best achieved with additional help by directed suprapubic pressure.

DELIVERY OF THE POSTERIOR ARM

This will succeed in the vast majority of cases, except in those rare instances of bilateral shoulder dystocia where the posterior shoulder has not entered the sacral bay. It is performed by passing the hand deep into the vagina along the fetal humerus to the elbow. In theory, pressure on the antecubital fossa will assist flexion of the forearm (Pinard's manoeuvre). In practice, this is not always so and one has to reach for the forearm, grasp the hand and wrist, and deliver the posterior arm across the fetal chest. The anterior shoulder may now be accessible. If not, support the fetal head and rotate the trunk and posterior shoulder 180 degrees, at which point the former anterior shoulder should rotate below the pelvic brim into the sacral bay and be accessible. Delivery of the posterior arm is one of the manoeuvres most likely to cause fracture of the clavicle and humerus. However, these injuries heal well without long-term disability.

ALL-FOURS MANOEUVRE

In this manoeuvre, the woman is guided to the all-fours position on her hands and knees. In this posture, gravity may help push the posterior shoulder forward and over the sacral promontory. In addition, the flexibility of the sacroiliac joints may cause a 1–2 cm increase in the anteroposterior diameter of the pelvic inlet. In this position, it is the posterior shoulder that is delivered first by gentle head traction. This technique was originally observed by an American midwife working with indigenous midwives in Guatemala (Meenan *et al.* 1991). There is a reported success rate of over 80% with this manoeuvre (Bruner *et al.* 1998). Assisting a woman with epidural analgesia into this position will require a number of personnel. Although experience with this manoeuvre is limited, the rationale and early reports suggest that it is worthwhile.

CEPHALIC REPLACEMENT

This procedure may have application in those rare cases of bilateral shoulder dystocia with both shoulders above the pelvic brim and inaccessible to other vaginal manoeuvres. The mechanism of delivery is reversed by grasping the fetal head in the hand, flexing it and returning it to the vagina. In many cases, this is apparently accomplished with greater ease than one would expect. On other occasions, uterine relaxation may have to be provided using glyceryl trinitrate or terbutaline. The fetal heart is monitored while preparations are made to deliver the infant by caesarean section. Cases have been recorded where more than an hour has elapsed between replacement of the head, followed by normal fetal heart recording and safe delivery by caesarean section (Sandberg 1985). The success rate reported is in excess of 90% but there is significant associated maternal morbidity, with ruptured uterus in some 5% and blood transfusion in 10%. Perinatal death and morbidity associated with asphyxia and brachial plexus palsy have occurred in a significant minority of the infants (O'Leary 1993; Sandberg 1999).

Although cephalic replacement and subsequent caesarean section seems a radical procedure, experience is accumulating that suggests it is worthwhile in those rare cases of shoulder dystocia in which the more standard manoeuvres to achieve vaginal delivery are unsuccessful.

ABDOMINAL RESCUE

Rare cases of so-called abdominal rescue have been described following failed cephalic replacement. If the head cannot be replaced vaginally high enough to allow its delivery by caesarean section, the lower segment uterine incision is made and, by direct manipulation, the anterior shoulder 'pops up', allowing descent of the posterior shoulder and direct rotation of the anterior shoulder to the oblique diameter so that the posterior shoulder now becomes accessible for manoeuvres to allow vaginal delivery of the infant (O'Leary and Cuva 1992).

SYMPHYSIOTOMY

Although this procedure has been suggested for cases of shoulder dystocia that are refractory to other manoeuvres, there are no published series of its successful use for this purpose. One report of three cases from the USA showed poor infant outcome and significant maternal morbidity (Goodwin *et al.* 1997). Symphysiotomy continues to have a place in developing countries for carefully selected cases of cephalopelvic disproportion. Those experienced with the procedure can perform it under local anaesthetic in less than five minutes. While it has theoretical potential for the management of rare cases of shoulder dystocia, it is unlikely to gain acceptance in developed countries where experience with the procedure is limited or nonexistent.

CLEIDOTOMY

This is often quoted as an alternative procedure in cases of shoulder dystocia. However, the deliberate fracture or cutting of the clavicle is not easy to achieve in the term fetus. Furthermore, there is the potential for trauma to the subclavian vessels. Thus, this procedure, is really only considered for the fetus that is dead or has a lethal anomaly.

There are few more composure-testing moments in the life of the birth attendant than those spent dealing with shoulder dystocia. An understanding of the mechanisms involved and the manoeuvres necessary to overcome the dystocia is essential for all labour ward personnel. A clear plan and sequence of manoeuvres should be laid out and practised by all involved with the care of women in labour.

After a case of shoulder dystocia it is important, for clinical audit and medico-legal purposes, that the accoucheur clearly writes in the chart the type, timing, and sequence of manoeuvres used (Baskett 2002).

References

Al-Quattam MM, Al-Kharfy TM. (1996) Obstetric brachial plexus injury in subsequent delivery. *Ann Plast Surg* 37:545–8.

Allen RH, Bankoski BR, Butzin CA, Nagey DA. (1994) Comparing clinician-applied loads for routine, difficult, and shoulder dystocia deliveries. *Am J Obstet Gynecol* 171:1621–7.

Bager B. (1997) Perinatally acquired brachial plexus palsy: a persisting challenge. *Acta Paediatr* 86:1214–19.

Baskett TF. (2001) Prediction and management of shoulder dystocia. In: Bonnar J, editor. *Recent Advances in Obstetrics and Gynaecology Volume 21.* Edinburgh: Churchill Livingstone. p.45–54.

Baskett TF. (2002) Shoulder dystocia. *Clin Obstet Gynaecol* 16:57–68.

Baskett TF, Allen AC. (1995) Perinatal implications of shoulder dystocia. *Obstet Gynecol* 86:14–17.

Bruner JP, Drummond SB, Meenan AL, Gaskin IM. (1998) All-fours maneuver for reducing shoulder dystocia during labor. *J Reprod Med* 43:439–43.

CESDI (Confidential Enquiry into Stillbirths and Deaths in Infancy). *5th Annual Report*. London: Maternal and Child Health Research Consortium. p. 73–9.

Chauhan SP, Hendricks NW, Megann EF, Morrison JC, Kenney SP, Devoe LD. (1998) Limitations of clinical and sonographic estimates of birth weight: experience with 1034 parturitions. *Obstet Gynecol* 91:72–7.

Delpapa EH, Mueller-Heubach E. (1991) Pregnancy outcome following ultrasound diagnosis of macrosomia. *Obstet Gynecol* 78:340–3.

Eng GD, Binder H, Getson P, O'Donnell R. (1996) Obstetrical brachial plexus palsy outcome with conservative management. *Muscle Nerve* 19:884–91.

Flannelly G, Simm A. (1995) A study of delivery following shoulder dystocia. *British Congress of Obstetrics and Gynaecology, Dublin, 4–7 July 1995. Abstracts.* London: Royal College of Obstetricians and Gynaecologists. Abstract 516.

Ginsberg NA, Moisidis C. (2001) How to predict recurrent shoulder dystocia. *Am J Obstet Gynecol* 184:1427–30.

Gonik B, Stringer CA, Held B. (1983) An alternative maneuver for management of shoulder dystocia. *Am J Obstet Gynecol* 145:882–4.

Gonik B, Allen R, Sorab J. (1989) Objective evaluation of the shoulder dystocia phenomenon: effects of maternal pelvic orientation on force reduction. *Obstet Gynecol* 74:44–8.

Goodwin TM, Banks E, Miller LK, Phalen JP. (1997) Catastrophic shoulder dystocia and emergency symphysiotomy. *Am J Obstet Gynecol* 177:463–4.

Leigh TH, James CE. (1998) Medico-legal commentary: shoulder dystocia. *Br J Obstet Gynaecol* 105:815–17.

Lewis DF, Raymond RC, Perkins MB. (1995) Recurrence rate of shoulder dystocia. *Am J Obstet Gynecol* 172:1369–71.

Meenan AL, Gaskin IM, Hunt P, Ball CA. (1991) A new (old) maneuver for the management of shoulder dystocia. *J Fam Pract* 32:625–9.

O'Leary J. (1993) Cephalic replacement for shoulder dystocia: present status and future role of the Zavanelli maneuver. *Obstet Gynecol* 82:847–50.

O'Leary JA, Cuva A. (1992) Abdominal rescue after failed cephalic replacement. *Obstet Gynecol* 80:514–16.

Olugbile A, Mascarenhas L. (2000) Review of shoulder dystocia at the Birmingham Women's Hospital. *J Obstet Gynaecol* 20:267–70.

Pollack RN, Buchman AS, Yaffe H, Divon MY. (2000) Obstetrical brachial palsy: pathogenesis, risk factors, and prevention. *Clin Obstet Gynecol* 43:236–46.

Rouse DJ, Owen J, Goldenberg RL, Cliver SP. (1996) The effectiveness and costs of elective cesarean section for fetal macrosomia diagnosed by ultrasound. *JAMA* 276;1490–6.

Rubin A. (1964) Management of shoulder dystocia. *JAMA* 189:835–7.

Sandberg E. (1985) The Zavanelli maneuver: a potentially revolutionary method for the resolution of shoulder dystocia. *Am J Obstet Gynecol* 152:479–84.

Sandberg EC. (1999) Zavanelli maneuver, twelve years of recorded experience. *Obstet Gynecol* 93:312–17.

Sherman DJ, Arieli S, Tovbin J, Siegel G, Caspi E, Bukovsky I. (1998) A comparison of clinical and ultrasonic estimation of fetal weight. *Obstet Gynecol* 91:212–17.

Smith RB, Lance C, Pearson JF. (1994) Shoulder dystocia: what happens at the next delivery? *Br J Obstet Gynaecol* 101:713–15.

Spong CY, Beall M, Rodrigues D, Ross MG. (1995) An objective definition of shoulder dystocia: prolonged head-to-body delivery intervals and/or the use of ancillary obstetric maneuvers. *Obstet Gynecol* 86:433–41.

Verspyck E, Goffinet F, Hellot MF, Milliez J, Marpau L. (1999) Newborn shoulder width: a prospective study of 2222 consecutive measurements. *Br J Obstet Gynaecol* 106:589–93.

Walle T, Hartikainen-Sorie AL. (1993) Obstetric shoulder injury: associated risk factors, prediction, and prognosis. *Acta Obstet Gynecol Scand* 72:450–4.

Wood C, Ng K, Houndslow D, Benning H. (1973) Time: an important variable in normal delivery. *J Obstet Gynaecol Br Cwlth* 80:295–8.

Woods CE. (1943) A principle of physics as applicable to shoulder delivery. *Am J Obstet Gynecol* 45:796–805.

14 Cord prolapse

Cord prolapse is the quintessential obstetric emergency. It occurs when part of the umbilical cord descends below the fetal presenting part. If the membranes are intact the condition is called cord presentation. The frequency range is about one in 200 to one in 600 deliveries. The fetal risk is hypoxia due to physical compression of the umbilical cord vessels between the fetal presenting part and maternal tissues or spasm of the vessels due to the colder temperature, should the cord prolapse through the introitus.

Aetiology

FACTORS THAT PREDISPOSE TO CORD PROLAPSE

- **Fetal**
  Prematurity and low birthweight
  Malpresentation
  Anomaly
  Multiple pregnancy
- **Placental**
  Polyhydramnios
  Minor degree of placenta praevia
- **Maternal**
  Pelvic tumours, e.g. cervical fibroid
  Pelvic contraction
  Rupture of membranes: spontaneous and amniotomy
  Obstetric manoeuvres: rotation of fetal head, version.

From the list of factors that predispose to cord prolapse it can be seen that anything that impedes the close application of the presenting part to the lower uterine segment and cervix will increase the likelihood of cord prolapse. Many of these factors are interrelated, such as the premature fetus, malpresentation, multiple pregnancy and polyhydramnios (Woo *et al.* 1983; Koonings *et al.* 1990; Critchlow *et al.* 1994).

The potential for amniotomy to cause cord prolapse is often cited. However, studies have not shown an increased risk of cord prolapse with amniotomy compared with spontaneous rupture of the membranes (Yla-Outinen *et al.* 1985; Roberts *et al.* 1997). With a prudent approach to amniotomy for both induction and augmentation of labour this need not lead to an increased risk of cord prolapse. Indeed, should prolapse of the cord occur at the time of amniotomy it is more likely to be diagnosed and dealt with promptly, compared with that occurring at the time of spontaneous rupture of the membranes.

By far the most common predisposing factors are the preterm low birthweight infant, malpresentation and multiple pregnancy.

Diagnosis

The clinical spectrum of umbilical cord prolapse may vary from the dramatic loop of cord outside the introitus to the more subtle, barely palpable, cord at the side and just below the presenting part. The diagnosis is usually made by vaginal examination, which should be carried out to exclude cord prolapse in all cases with specific fetal heart rate abnormalities in labour (e.g. bradycardia or marked variable decelerations) and after spontaneous rupture of the membranes associated with breech presentation or a high presenting part.

Cord presentation is a much rarer diagnosis, which is sometimes made with a loop of cord felt through the membranes and below the presenting part or using ultrasound before the onset or during early labour (Jones *et al.* 2000).

Management

Speed is of the essence and the perinatal outcome is largely dictated by the diagnosis–delivery interval (Katz *et al.* 1988; Murphy and Mackenzie 1995). The three components of management are:

- prevent or relieve cord compression and cord artery spasm
- fetal assessment
- prompt delivery of the infant (Prabulos and Philipson 1998).

PREVENT OR RELIEVE CORD COMPRESSION AND CORD ARTERY SPASM

This is the essential first line of treatment. If the cord has prolapsed outside the introitus, the umbilical circulation is compromised by spasm of the umbilical vessels due to the colder temperature. The cord should be cradled gently in the hand and replaced as high as possible in the vagina. Careful handling of the cord is necessary, as even light trauma may also cause spasm of the vessels. When the cord has been replaced in the vagina or if the cord has only prolapsed within the vagina, the entire cord should be cradled in the palm of the hand in such a manner that the compression forces of the vagina are relieved. The tips of the fingers can be used to elevate the presenting part so that it does not directly compress the cord, but not so much as to cause further cord prolapse. An alternative is to place a Foley catheter in the bladder and fill to approximately 500 ml, which should assist in elevating the presenting part and prevent cord compression (Chetty and Moodley 1980; Runnebaum and Katz 1999). Intravenous tocolytic treatment may have rare application when delay is incurred.

If possible, the bed should be put in the Trendelenburg position. Initially, the mother should be placed in the knee–chest position, which gives maximum elevation of the presenting part. If there is any delay this is too tiring a position to maintain and the woman can be moved to the lateral Sims position with the buttocks elevated by pillows.

If facilities for anaesthesia and caesarean section are not immediately available then the above tactics must be maintained and have, on occasions, been applied successfully for several hours. In these cases, the Sims lateral position with elevated hips is the most comfortable for the woman.

Very rarely, with minor degrees of cord prolapse, it is possible to replace the cord above the presenting part and allow labour to continue. Occasionally this is easily achieved, but it is not appropriate to attempt much manipulation as it risks trauma and prolonged vascular spasm of the cord.

FETAL ASSESSMENT

While cord compression is being relieved, urgent attention should be directed to assessing the fetus. If the fetus is dead, immature or has a lethal anomaly then immediate caesarean section is obviously contraindicated. In many cases the antenatal record will provide the information on gestation and the presence or absence of a lethal anomaly. If the patient has no antenatal record, a clinical estimate will have to be made of the size and viability of the infant. Whether or not the fetus is alive is best determined by listening to the fetal heart rate and/or palpating the umbilical artery pulsations. On occasion this can be quite difficult and maternal soft tissue pulsations may be detectable. In addition, the clinician has often been summoned at speed to the labour ward and arrives in a hyperdynamic state, so that pulsations in their own fingers may be confusing. If there are no detectable pulsations in the cord, a scalp electrode may be of assistance, particularly in monitoring the fetus during the delay between diagnosis and delivery. If available, real-time ultrasound of the fetal chest should confirm the presence or absence of fetal heart activity. This may be present even in the absence of umbilical artery pulsations and the procedure should be performed before abandoning the fetus without detectable cord pulsation (Driscoll *et al.* 1987).

DELIVERY

In most cases the fetus should be delivered by immediate caesarean section. The person whose hand is cradling the cord and elevating the presenting part may remain in position during the induction of anaesthesia and the placement of sterile sheets. If the full-bladder technique has been used the Foley catheter is drained at this point – if not, a catheter is inserted. Once the caesarean section is underway and as the surgeon approaches the lower segment incision, a warning can be issued to remove the protective hand from the surgical site.

On rare occasions the cervix is fully dilated and the presenting part low in the pelvis together with the prolapsed cord. In these cases rapid assisted vaginal delivery will be the choice. Depending on the circumstances this may involve delivery by forceps, vacuum or breech extraction.

If the fetus is dead, immature or has a lethal anomaly, then caesarean section would only be carried out for maternal reasons – such as an obstructed labour with a transverse lie – that cannot be resolved safely by vaginal manipulation and delivery.

It is emphasised that in the vast majority of cases the calm and orderly application of the above principles will result in safe delivery of the infant.

References

Chetty RM, Moodley J. (1980) Umbilical cord prolapse. *S Afr Med J* 57:128–9.

Critchlow CW, Leet TL, Benedetti TJ, Daling JR. (1994) Risk factors and infant outcomes associated with umbilical cord prolapse: a population-based case–control study among births in Washington State. *Am J Obstet Gynecol* 170:613–8.

Driscoll JA, Sadan O, Van Gelderen CJ, Holloway GA. (1987) Cord prolapse – can we save more babies? *Br J Obstet Gynaecol* 1987;94:594–5.

Jones G, Grenier S, Gruslin A. (2000) Sonographic diagnosis of funic presentation: implications for delivery. *Br J Obstet Gynaecol* 107:1055–7.

Katz Z. Shoham Z, Lancet M, Blickstein I, Mogilner BM, Zalel Y. (1988) Management of labor with umbilical cord prolapse: a 5-year study. *Obstet Gynecol* 72:278–80.

Koonings PP, Paul RH, Campbell K. (1990) Umbilical cord prolapse: a contemporary look. *J Reprod Med* 35:690–2.

Murphy DJ, Mackenzie IZ. (1995) The mortality and morbidity associated with umbilical cord prolapse. *Br J Obstet Gynaecol* 102:826–30.

Prabulos AM, Philipson EH. (1998) Umbilical cord prolapse: Is the time from diagnosis to delivery critical? *J Reprod Med* 43:129–32.

Roberts WE, Martin RW, Roach HH, Perry KG, Martin JN, Morrison JC. (1997) Are obstetric interventions such as cervical ripening, induction of labor, amnioinfusion or amniotomy associated with umbilical cord prolapse? *Am J Obstet Gynecol* 176:1181–3.

Runnebaum IB, Katz M. (1999) Intrauterine resuscitation by rapid urinary bladder instillation in a case of occult prolapse of an excessively long umbilical cord. *Eur J Obstet Gynecol Reprod Biol* 84:101–2.

Woo JSK, Ngan YS, Ma HK. (1983) Prolapse and presentation of the umbilical cord. *Aust N Z J Obstet Gynaecol* 23:142–5.

Yla-Outinen, Heinonen P K, Tuimala R. (1985) Predisposing and risk factors of umbilical cord prolapse. *Acta Obstet Gynecol Scand* 64:567–70.

15 Antepartum haemorrhage

Antepartum haemorrhage is bleeding from the genital tract from 20 weeks of gestation until delivery of the baby. This definition may vary from 20 to 24 weeks of gestation in different countries, in keeping with local medical and legal definitions of fetal viability.

The main causes are: placenta praevia (one in 200–250), placental abruption (one in 150) and unclassified (one in 100). At times, women in preterm labour may present with bleeding. In addition, a number of patients present with antepartum bleeding from lower genital tract lesions such as vulvovaginal varices, cervical polyp and cervical cancer. While these are important to diagnose and treat they will not, as a group, be considered further in this chapter.

Placenta praevia

In this condition the placenta is implanted in part or in whole on the lower uterine segment, which is that portion of the uterus beneath the reflection of the uterovesical peritoneum. Functionally it is that part of the uterine muscle that develops in the latter half of pregnancy, is stretched and thinned during late pregnancy and is relatively passive and non-contractile. When fully developed in labour it may extend 7–8 cm from the internal os.

The incidence of placenta praevia is increased with higher parity, advancing maternal age and particularly in those previously delivered by caesarean section. The overall recurrence risk of placenta praevia is approximately one in 20.

Types I and II constitute a minor degree and types III and IV a major degree of placenta praevia. Approximately 50% of all cases of placenta praevia are minor and 50% are major (Figure 15.1).

CLINICAL FEATURES

In the later weeks of pregnancy and during labour the lower uterine segment is progressively stretched and thinned. It is therefore common for that part of the placenta implanted on the lower uterine segment to

CLASSIFICATION AND TERMINOLOGY OF THE TYPES OR DEGREES OF PLACENTA PRAEVIA

- Type I (lateral or low-lying)
  Extends onto the lower uterine segment but not as far as the edge of the internal os.
- Type II (marginal)
  The edge of the placenta extends down to the internal os but does not cover it.
- Type III (partial)
  The edge of the placenta covers the internal os but only partially when it is dilated.
- Type IV (complete or central)
  The placenta completely covers the cervix even at full dilatation.

separate and cause bleeding. In 70–80% of cases this bleeding will occur before the onset of labour. In general, the more major the degree of praevia the earlier and heavier the bleeding, although some minor degrees can be just as treacherous. As the bleeding comes from the placental site in the lower uterine segment there is minimal resistance to the blood passing through the cervix and, thus, little or no extravasation of blood into the uterine muscle, resulting in painless bleeding. As a result, the uterus is usually soft and not tender and the patient's haemodynamic status corresponds to the apparent blood loss. In contrast to placental abruption, the fetus is rarely threatened by placenta praevia, particularly

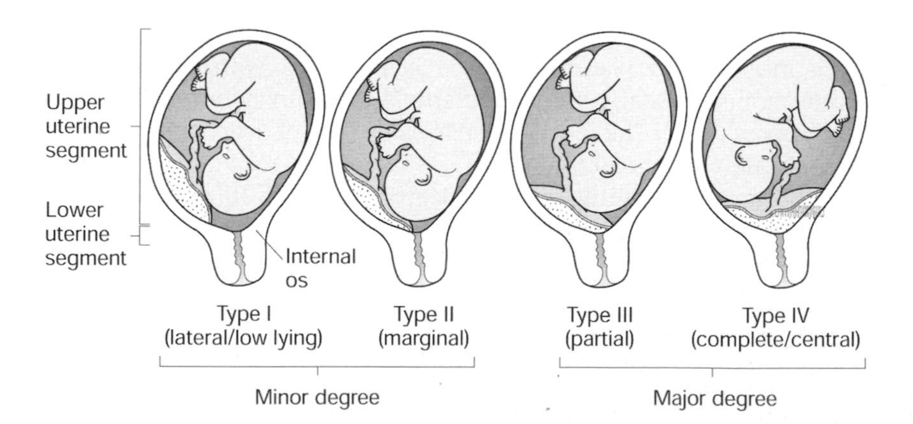

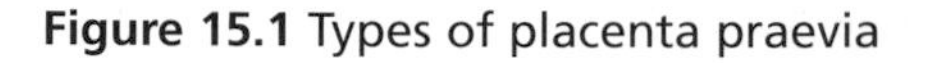
Figure 15.1 Types of placenta praevia

Table 15.1 Clinical features of placental abruption and placenta praevia (reproduced with permission from Baskett TF. (1999) *Essential Management of Obstetric Emergencies*. 3rd ed. Clinical Press Ltd. p. 65)

Placental abruption	*Placenta praevia*
May be associated with hypertensive disorders, uterine overdistension, trauma	Apparently causeless
Abdominal pain and/or backache	Painless
Uterine tenderness	Uterus not tender
Increased uterine tone	Uterus soft
Usually normal presentation	Malpresentation and/or high presenting part
Fetal heart may be absent	Fetal heart usually normal
Shock and anaemia out of proportion to apparent blood loss	Shock and anaemia correspond to apparent blood loss

with the first bleed. With the placenta occupying part or all of the lower uterine segment the presenting part of the fetus is more commonly high and free, with malpresentation such as breech, transverse or unstable lie being found in about 40% of cases.

The distinguishing clinical features between placenta praevia and placental abruption are shown in Table 15.1.

DIAGNOSIS

Ultrasound is the technique of choice. However, early in the second trimester when most screening ultrasounds are performed, the lower uterine segment is unformed and extends only 0.5 cm from the internal os. Thus, a false diagnosis of low-lying placenta is commonly made at this stage. With transabdominal ultrasound this may occur in 5–20% of cases, although transvaginal ultrasound has improved considerably upon this level of accuracy. Furthermore, transvaginal ultrasound has not been found to increase the risk of haemorrhage. If an ultrasound diagnosis of possible placenta praevia is made in the second trimester in an asymptomatic patient, it should be repeated at 32–34 weeks of gestation when the lower segment is formed and the true position of the placenta can be delineated.

The ultimate confirmation of the diagnosis is to feel the placenta with the examining finger placed through the cervix. Such examination is only done under planned, double set-up conditions (see later). With the accuracy of transvaginal ultrasound this is now rarely used, although it may have occasional application under certain circumstances (see later).

MANAGEMENT

If the patient has an ultrasound suggesting placenta praevia in the second trimester but no bleeding, a repeat ultrasound is planned for 32–34 weeks of gestation to delineate the true site of the placenta (see above). In the vast majority of cases the placenta, thought to be low lying in the second trimester, will be shown not to be so.

If, at 32–34 weeks of gestation, a transvaginal ultrasound continues to show a minor degree of placenta praevia, then the patient should be advised of this and warned to avoid vaginal intercourse, limit her travel and have a mechanism for seeking immediate attention if vaginal bleeding occurs. If no bleeding occurs, she may be managed as an outpatient until 36–38 weeks of gestation and a repeat ultrasound performed. At this point, she should be admitted for delivery, which may be by elective caesarean section if the placenta praevia is of a major degree and the level of ultrasound in the institution is secure. If there is any doubt or it is a minor degree of anterior praevia, examination in the operating theatre should be arranged to confirm or deny the diagnosis (see later).

The asymptomatic woman who has a major degree of placenta praevia at the 32–34-week ultrasound should be admitted to hospital for the remainder of her pregnancy.

The woman who has an antepartum bleed should be admitted, have an intravenous infusion established with crystalloid and blood taken for group, screen and crossmatch. Clinical assessment may then point to the likelihood of placenta praevia or placental abruption. Provided that the bleeding is not of a magnitude that requires immediate intervention ultrasound can be arranged to confirm or deny the diagnosis of placenta praevia. In general, the first bleed associated with placenta praevia settles spontaneously and is not threatening to either the mother or the fetus. If it occurs before the onset of labour and before 37–38 weeks of gestation, provided it settles, expectant management is undertaken. This entails keeping the woman in hospital, seeking and treating anaemia and, in selected cases, performing a speculum examination to rule out concomitant lower genital tract lesions. If the patient is rhesus (Rh) negative, Rh immune globulin should be given and a Kleihauer test performed to ensure that an adequate dose has been given to cover any fetomaternal bleed. The patient is initially treated with bed rest and bathroom privileges and then allowed more freedom in the ward. In those cases under 34 weeks, steroids to mature the fetal lungs should be considered in case early intervention is necessary.

The cost for the health service and the disruption to the patient and her family of admission to hospital, potentially for several weeks, is considerable. There is controversy as to whether all patients with a confirmed diagnosis of placenta praevia should remain in hospital or whether this can be on a selective basis (Droste and Liel 1994; Mouer 1994; Wing *et al.* 1996). There are no unequivocal data upon which to base this decision. However, in general, those women who have a placenta praevia and bleed before the onset of labour have a worse perinatal outcome than those who do not bleed (Rosen and Peek 1994; Love and Wallace 1996; Lamb *et al.* 2000). Thus, if one is going to be selective in admitting patients with placenta praevia, those who have bled should be admitted.

If the patient has reached 37–38 weeks of gestation, if labour is established or if they continue to bleed, active management in the form of delivery is indicated. If the accuracy of ultrasound in the hospital is unequivocal this will be by caesarean section. If the level of ultrasound is not secure or, in parts of the world where ultrasound may not be available, the so-called double set-up examination in the operating theatre may be necessary. This entails availability of anaesthesia, nursing personnel and equipment immediately prepared to move straight to caesarean section should the presence of placenta praevia be confirmed by gentle digital examination. First the head should be palpated through the fornices and if felt the finger is gently passed through the cervix. If the placenta is not found to encroach upon the lower uterine segment by the examining finger then amniotomy and careful monitoring of the subsequent labour may be appropriate.

In general, all cases of confirmed placenta praevia are now treated by caesarean section. One can make an argument, in the most minor degree of praevia in which the presenting part has settled past the bleeding edge of the placenta and all other aspects are favourable, for amniotomy and careful monitoring of the induced labour. However, in all but these few cases caesarean section is more appropriate.

TECHNICAL ASPECTS OF CAESAREAN SECTION FOR PLACENTA PRAEVIA

In most cases the lower uterine segment is sufficiently developed to allow a low transverse incision to be made. Often, there are enlarged vessels over the lower uterus, However, provided that the lower segment is well developed this should not deter one from using the transverse incision. If the lower segment is marginally developed and there are large vessels at the lateral margins then classical caesarean section may be the safer option.

Once the uterine incision has been made in the usual fashion it is best to go to the edge of the placenta, rupture the membranes and bring the presenting part through the incision. Scrutiny of the ultrasound before the operation should guide the direction, whether this is up, down or lateral, to gain access to the membranes. This is much better than cutting through the placenta, which increases the risk of fetal exsanguination.

Because the lower uterine segment is much less contractile than the upper segment, bleeding from the placenta site in this area is common. A number of techniques can be used to try and overcome haemorrhage from the placental site.

- Firm packing of the lower uterine segment for five minutes will often reduce the bleeding completely or help delineate specific bleeding sites that can be oversewn with figure-of-eight sutures. Alternatively, square sutures going through the entire thickness of the uterine wall may help stem oozing areas (Cho *et al.* 2000). Sub-endomyometrial injection at multiple sites, each of 1–2 ml solution of vasopressin (5 units in 20 ml saline), has been recorded as effective in some cases (Lurie *et al.* 1996).
- If conservation of the uterus is strongly desired, both uterine arteries can be ligated, although this may not sufficiently reduce the blood supply to the area of the internal os. Another option is to provide tamponade with a balloon device or packing and bring this out through the cervix and vagina. The lower uterine segment is then sewn over this pack. This may be effective when the upper uterine segment is well contracted and the bleeding is coming purely from the placental site in the lower segment. Such treatment may also allow one to buy time to marshal the resources for uterine artery embolisation.
- If the above is unsuccessful, and particularly if the patient's family is complete, then total abdominal hysterectomy should be definitive. In this instance, subtotal hysterectomy may fail to stem the bleeding from the residual cervix.
- If there is placenta praevia accreta hysterectomy will almost always be required. When placenta praevia accreta is known to exist or is highly likely before the caesarean section is undertaken, it has been suggested that pre-operative placement of vascular catheters in the internal iliac arteries may allow one to embolise the vessels, contain the haemorrhage and preserve the uterus (Hansch *et al.* 1999).

Caesarean section for placenta praevia, with or without accreta, is not a procedure for the inexperienced. In cases in which the likelihood of placenta praevia accreta is high, based on clinical, ultrasound or MRI findings, the possibility of caesarean hysterectomy should be discussed beforehand with the woman. Senior and experienced staff must be present for these cases in which the haemorrhage can be massive and unrelenting.

VAGINAL DELIVERY WITH PLACENTA PRAEVIA

There may be rare occasions, such as intrauterine death, lethal anomaly, extreme prematurity or lack of appropriate hospital facilities when the largely historical techniques of assisted vaginal delivery may be appropriate. These include Braxton Hicks bipolar podalic version, which involves the external hand guiding the breech over the pelvic brim and two fingers of the internal hand pushed through the cervix to grasp a foot and pull it through the membranes and cervix. In this manner, the fetal buttock acts by tamponade on the placenta and the bleeding lower uterine site. This can be a very effective haemostat. The fetus is not forcibly pulled through the cervix but steady gentle traction is applied to the foot to achieve tamponade and actively promote progressive dilatation of the cervix (Lawson *et al.* 2001).

Should the fetus present by the head, Willett's scalp forceps can be applied to the fetal scalp through the incompletely dilated cervix and with traction, apply tamponade and assisted delivery in a similar manner. These techniques are very rarely indicated but worth keeping in mind for the rare case of a dead or nonviable fetus or in places with inadequate facilities for caesarean section (Baskett 2001).

Vasa praevia

Vasa praevia is an uncommon but potentially disastrous complication occurring in about one in 5000 deliveries. It is associated with velamentous insertion of the cord, in which the site of umbilical cord insertion is into the membranes rather than directly into the placenta. Thus, the umbilical vessels pass between the membranes, unsupported by Wharton's jelly, before running into the placenta. As such these vessels are very vulnerable to compression and tearing. When the vessels of velamentous insertion run across the lower segment and cervix in front of the presenting part, vasa praevia exists.

These vessels may be compressed as the fetal presenting part descends or, more commonly, be torn when the membranes rupture either spontaneously or by amniotomy.

On rare occasions, the vessels can be felt by the astute examiner during pelvic assessment. Ultrasound Doppler colour flow has been used to demonstrate vasa praevia on rare occasions. Usually, however, the first manifestation is vaginal bleeding and fetal heart rate abnormalities just after rupture of the membranes. In these circumstances, immediate caesarean section is indicated but is often too late to avoid fetal exsanguination.

Placental abruption

Placental abruption is the partial or complete premature separation of a normally situated placenta before the birth of the fetus. In the older literature it was called 'accidental' haemorrhage to distinguish it from the 'inevitable' haemorrhage of placenta praevia.

CAUSES

In most cases the cause of placental abruption is unknown. There are a number of non-specific associations including:

- high parity
- increased maternal age
- smoking
- cocaine use
- low socio-economic group
- hypertensive disorders
- Sudden decompression of an overdistended uterus, such as follows rupture of the membranes with polyhydramnios or after delivery of the first twin
- Prolonged prelabour rupture of the membranes
- Circumvallate placenta
- Trauma, such as a fall, car accident or amniocentesis, is an uncommon cause.

TYPES OF ABRUPTION (FIGURE 15.2)

- **Revealed haemorrhage**
  Occurs when the edge of the placenta separates so there is little resistance to the blood tracking down between the membranes and the uterine wall to pass through the cervix.
- **Concealed haemorrhage**
  Much less frequent and occurs when the blood is trapped between the placenta and uterine wall and does not appear externally.
- **Mixed haemorrhage**
  Occurs when there is a degree of both the above types.
  In addition to the above classification and depending on the amount of blood loss and the severity of the signs and symptoms, cases may be defined as mild, moderate or severe.

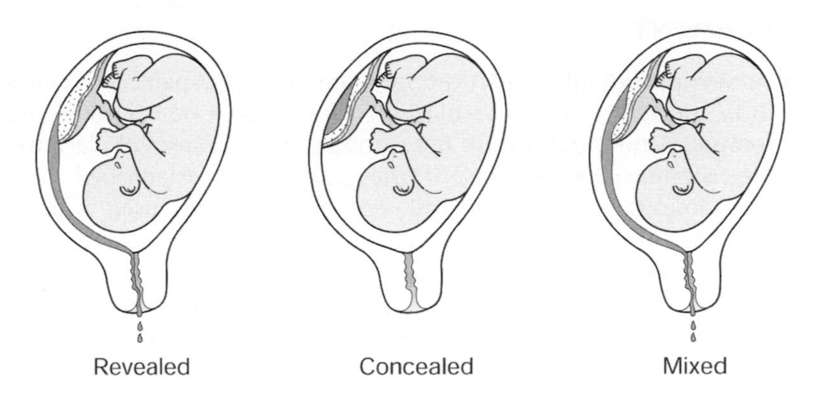

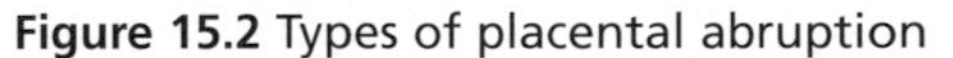

Figure 15.2 Types of placental abruption

PATHOPHYSIOLOGY AND CLINICAL FEATURES

Haemorrhage occurs into the decidua basalis. If this bleeding is at the periphery of the placenta then the blood will track down with minimal resistance between the membranes and uterine wall and be revealed. Because there is little extravasation into the myometrium there may be minimal pain or uterine irritability and tenderness. Thus, these mild revealed cases may mimic placenta praevia. At the other extreme, the bleeding may be located more centrally and be concealed. There is retroplacental haematoma formation and, as the blood is under pressure, it may extravasate to varying degrees into the myometrium. This will increase the uterine tone, irritability and pain, probably due to prostaglandin release from the damaged decidual tissue. Labour often ensues. If the blood dissects through the myometrium to the subserosal surface of the uterus, this discolouration can be seen at the time of caesarean section and is known as Couvelaire uterus. In the severe concealed case, there is unremitting abdominal pain and the uterus is hard and tender. The fetus dies. Decidual thromboplastins may be forced into the maternal circulation and initiate disseminated intravascular coagulation. Together with hypovolaemic shock, there is intense vasoconstriction and if this causes prolonged renal arteriolar spasm it may lead to tubular and cortical necrosis and, ultimately, renal failure. In between these two extreme clinical pictures cases of mixed haemorrhage will occur.

The clinical hallmarks of placental abruption are abdominal pain, increased uterine tone and tenderness, hypovolaemic shock out of proportion to the apparent blood loss and, in the more severe cases, fetal death.

MANAGEMENT

The recumbent pregnant woman can maintain a normal pulse and blood pressure in the face of considerable blood loss (up to one-third of the blood volume). Under-transfusion is a common error in cases of placental abruption (Bonnar 2000). Thus, if the diagnosis is established, two intravenous lines should be set up and crystalloid rapidly infused. At least four units of blood should be crossmatched. In moderate and severe cases, blood transfusion will be required. A working guide to the adequacy of circulation is to keep the haematocrit above 30% and the urinary output greater than 30 ml per hour. In severe cases, central venous pressure monitoring, if available, will guide transfusion. The management of disseminated intravascular coagulation is outlined in Chapter 16.

Obstetric management will vary with the type and severity of placental abruption.

- In mild revealed cases, with no uterine tenderness, expectant treatment may be followed until 37–40 weeks of gestation, when induction of labour is undertaken based on the timing and amount of blood loss.
- If the diagnosis of placental abruption is certain and the fetus is mature and alive, steps should be taken to expedite delivery. It is not uncommon for patients to already be in early labour when the diagnosis is established. If so, amniotomy is advisable, as this will reduce the intrauterine pressure and, at least theoretically, reduce the risk of extravasation of blood and thromboplastins into the myometrium and maternal circulation. If the fetus is already dead, the labour usually progresses rapidly to spontaneous delivery. If labour progress is inadequate, oxytocin augmentation is appropriate. If the fetus is alive and the clinical signs are mild, the fetal heart may be monitored to anticipate vaginal delivery.
- Caesarean section is used liberally for moderate and severe cases, when the fetus is mature and alive, in cases unfavourable for induction of labour, if there is significant bleeding, and those in whom there is poor progress of labour after six to eight hours.

Unclassified antepartum haemorrhage

In about 50% of cases of antepartum haemorrhage the diagnosis of placenta praevia or placental abruption cannot be established, even after delivery. Such cases are therefore called unclassified or of unknown origin. Some of these are minor degrees of placenta praevia and placental abruption that cannot be confirmed. Others are probably due to disruption of small vessels in the cervix during formation of the lower uterine segment. These are usually cases of mild bleeding that are treated expectantly and ultrasound shows no evidence of placenta praevia and there are no clinical signs of placental abruption. After initial assessment these patients can be treated outside hospital, but fetal growth and wellbeing should be followed as perinatal loss is increased in this group as a whole. Induction of labour at or close to term should be considered.

References

Baskett TF. (2001) Of violent floodings in pregnancy: evolution of the management of placenta praevia. In: Sturdee D, Oláh K, Keane D, editors. *Yearbook of Obstetrics and Gynaecology Volume 9*. London: RCOG Press. p. 1–14.

Bonnar J. (2000) Massive obstetric haemorrhage. *Clin Obstet Gynaecol* 14:1–18.

Cho JH, Jun HS, Lee CN. (2000) Hemostatic suturing technique for uterine bleeding during cesarean delivery. *Obstet Gynecol* 96:129–31.

Droste S, Kiel K. (1994) Expectant management of placenta previa: cost-benefit analysis of outpatient treatment. *Am J Obstet Gynecol* 170:1254–7.

Hansch E, Chitkara U, McAlpine J, El-Sayed Y, Dake MD, Razavi MK. (1999) Pelvic artery embolization for control of obstetric hemorrhage: a five year experience. *Am J Obstet Gynecol* 180:1454–9.

Hassim AM. (2001) Obstetric haemorrhage. In: Lawson JB, Harrison KA, Bergström S, editors. *Maternity Care in Developing Countries*. London: RCOG Press. p. 160–78.

Lamb CS, Wong SF, Chow KM, Ho LC. (2000) Women with placenta praevia and antepartum haemorrhage have a worse outcome than those who do not bleed before delivery. *J Obstet Gynaecol* 20:27–31.

Love CD, Wallace EM. (1996) Pregnancies complicated by placenta praevia: what is appropriate management? *Br J Obstet Gynaecol* 103:864–7.

Lurie S, Appleman Z, Katz Z. (1996) Intractable postpartum bleeding duc to placenta accreta: local vasopressin may save the uterus. *Br J Obstet Gynaecol* 103:1164.

Mouer JR. (1994) Placenta previa: antepartum conservative management, inpatient versus outpatient. *Am J Obstet Gynecol* 170:1683–6.

Rosen DM, Peek MJ. (1994) Do women with placenta praevia without antepartum haemorrhage require hospitalisation? *Aust N Z J Obstet Gynaecol* 34:130–4.

Wing DA, Paul RH, Millar LK. (1996) Management of the symptomatic placenta previa: a randomized, controlled trial of inpatient versus outpatient expectant management. *Am J Obstet Gynecol* 175:806–11.

Further reading

American College of Obstetricians and Gynecologists. (2002) *Placenta Accreta. Committee Opinion No. 266*. Washington DC: ACOG.

Royal College of Obstetricians and Gynaecologists. (2001) *Placenta Praevia: Diagnosis and Management. Guideline No. 27*. London: RCOG.

Hl-adky K, Yankowitz J, Hansen WF. Placental abruption (2002) *Obstet Gynecol Surv* 57:299–305.

16 Postpartum haemorrhage

Primary postpartum haemorrhage (PPH) is defined as bleeding from the genital tract in excess of 500 ml within 24 hours of delivery. The reported incidence varies from 2–10% because blood loss is such a subjective appraisal. It is a clinical truism that doctors underestimate blood loss while patients overestimate it. This is supported by blood volume studies, which show that the normal parturient loses about 500 ml at delivery. Thus, when the doctor estimates the patient has lost 500 ml they may have lost closer to one litre. Therefore, in terms of clinical management, the working definition of estimated 500 ml blood loss is a reasonable one. It is also advisable to have a lower tolerance for blood loss with small women, who have a smaller blood volume, and in those who are already anaemic. Because of the latter two factors some define PPH as a greater than 500 ml blood loss or that which causes haemodynamic changes.

Aetiology

Uterine atony is the cause in 80–85% of cases, due to a failure of or interference with the normal mechanisms that ensure the haemostatic contraction and retraction of the uterine musculature (see Chapter 4). This can occur in normal cases but is more often associated with:

- high parity
- overdistension of the uterus with multiple pregnancy, polyhydramnios and macrosomia
- prolonged, precipitate or induced labour are all more likely to be associated with uterine atony following delivery
- antepartum haemorrhage: both placenta praevia and placental abruption
- drugs: tocolytic agents and general anaesthesia with halothane
- retained placenta, placental fragments and blood clots (see Chapter 4)
- structural abnormalities of the uterus, such as uterine fibroids or anomalies, may interfere with uterine retraction
- mismanagement of the third stage with manipulation of the fundus

and premature cord traction can lead to partial separation of the placenta and increased blood loss.

Genital tract trauma is the second most common cause, accounting for 10–15% of cases:

- episiotomy
- lacerations of the perineum, vagina and cervix
- laceration or rupture of the uterus
- vulvovaginal and broad ligament haematomas.

Other causes are acute uterine inversion and disseminated intravascular coagulation.

Medical management

PREVENTION

The prevention of PPH by active management of the third stage of labour is discussed in Chapter 4.

OXYTOCIC DRUGS

The immediate management of atonic postpartum haemorrhage is to contract the uterus. The first thing to hand is, in fact, the hand and it should be used to apply vigorous but tender fundal massage.

The oxytocic drugs have been covered in detail in Chapter 4 but their application in the management of uterine atony will be covered here.

- Give intravenous oxytocin 5 units, or ergometrine 0.2 mg, intravenously. This can be repeated within a few minutes if required.
- 30–40 units of oxytocin in 500 ml crystalloid solution run in briskly to initiate and continue uterine contraction.

The above first-line oxytocic drugs will usually control most cases of atonic PPH. If not, one should not hesitate to move to the prostaglandins:

- 15-methyl prostaglandin F2α – carboprost – (Hemabate®, Pharmacia) 0.25 mg, is given by intramuscular or intramyometrial injection. This can be repeated several times in desperate cases.
- Although misoprostol is usually given orally and is absorbed quite quickly by this route, it is usually not the preferred method of administration in atonic PPH. Obviously, the vaginal route is impractical as it is rapidly washed out by the bleeding. Misoprostol has been given rectally in doses up to 1000 μg for atonic PPH (O'Brien *et al.* 1998).

- The uterus that is unresponsive to one oxytocic may respond to another, so there should be no delay in moving from one oxytocic drug to another. Carboprost has proved to be effective in many cases in which oxytocin and ergometrine have failed. In general, oxytocic drugs are more likely to fail in cases of prolonged labour with chorioamnionitis.

TREAT HYPOVOLAEMIA

With postpartum haemorrhage there should be early recourse to rapid intravenous infusion of crystalloid (Ringer-Lactate and physiological saline). Two intravenous lines of access should be established with 14–16-gauge cannulae – intravenous crystalloid can be infused twice as fast through a 14-gauge, compared with an 18-gauge cannula. In healthy women who are not anaemic, a blood loss of up to 1500 ml can usually be managed with rapid infusion of crystalloid. This assumes that the bleeding has been arrested. In the woman who is already anaemic, or in the patient who loses 2000 ml or more, transfusion of packed red cells will be necessary. If the blood loss is massive and the patient has hypovolaemic shock, both intravenous crystalloid and colloid, in the form of 5% albumin or a 5% protein solution (albumin 88%, alpha globulins 7% and beta globulins 5%; Plasmanate®, Bayer), will be required until blood is available. Fresh frozen plasma can be obtained quickly in many hospitals or, alternatively, 5% albumin, which is the colloid of choice, can be given. As albumin is very viscous, it should be drawn up with a wide-bore needle and added to physiological saline so that it can be rapidly infused.

CONTINUOUS FUNDAL MASSAGE

On rare occasions the uterus is unresponsive to oxytocic drugs but will contract with continuous uterine massage. This should be vigorous but not so hard as to cause trauma or pain to the patient. In cases with persistent ooze, the patient herself can be taught to massage her own uterine fundus.

BIMANUAL UTERINE COMPRESSION

The vaginal hand formed as a fist in the anterior fornix and the abdominal hand cupping and pushing down on the posterofundal part of the uterus may provide temporary compression and reduction of bleeding (Figure 16.1). In addition, rotary massage between the fist and hand may help to contract the uterus. This is painful and can only be used in the short term or in those with epidural analgesia.

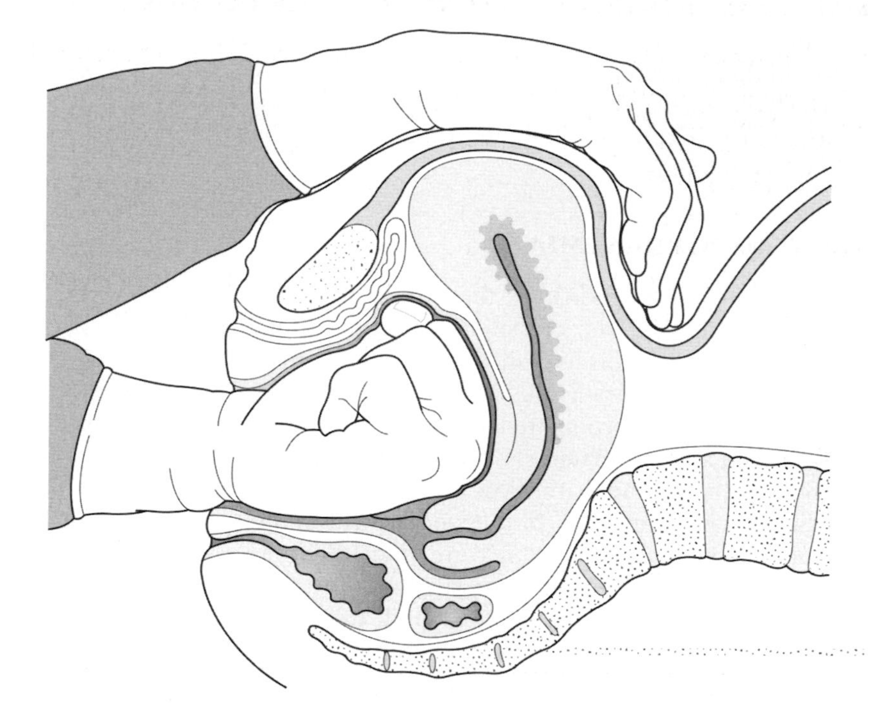

Figure 16.1 Bimanual compression of the uterus

AORTIC COMPRESSION

This is a fairly desperate move that may be tried in the thin patient. One hand pulls the uterine fundus out of the pelvis and pushes upwards and backwards across the lower part of the uterus, while the other hand directs the fundus posteriorly to compress the aorta.

The above three manoeuvres are generally used as temporary measures before moving to surgical options.

Surgical management

There are a number of surgical approaches that may be required for uterine or lower genital tract haemorrhage (Tamizian and Arulkumaran 2001).

SUTURE OF LOWER GENITAL TRACT LACERATIONS

Lower genital tract lacerations may bleed profusely and should be sutured with a continuous locking stitch. Adequate exposure, light and assistance are necessary for cervical and high-vaginal lacerations. It can be hard to identify the apex of these lacerations. This is best done by placing a suture as high as you can and using this as a tractor to bring the top of the laceration into view. At times it may be best to oversew each side of the vaginal laceration separately to control the bleeding. This avoids tearing through of the sutures and may prevent narrowing of the upper vagina. The space between the sutured edges heals well with time. Following suture it is often necessary to place a tight vaginal pack and a Foley catheter in the bladder.

CERVICAL LACERATIONS

Cervical lacerations can be identified with the use of two ring forceps. The anterior lip is grasped with one forcep and the second placed at 2–3 o'clock. In this way, the cervix between the two forceps can be carefully inspected. The forcep on the anterior lip is then removed and placed beyond the second forcep at 5–6 o'clock. This is done sequentially so that the entire cervical circumference is visualised. Small lacerations without bleeding need not be sutured. Larger lacerations, ≥ 3 cm or those that are bleeding, should be sutured with a continuous locking stitch. This is facilitated by placing ring forceps on either side of the laceration, both for haemostasis and to steady the tissues while suturing. The postpartum cervix is usually oedematous and friable and if, despite suturing, the cervix continues to ooze, the bleeding edges can be controlled by applying ring forceps and leaving them in place for a few hours. The patient is able to lie flat with these two ring forceps in place with minimal discomfort.

VULVAL AND PARAVAGINAL HAEMATOMAS

Vulval and paravaginal haematomas should be incised and clot evacuated. Seek and ligate active bleeding points. Often, no discreet bleeding points are found, but areas that are oozing should be oversewn. Following incision, evacuation and suture, the vagina should be tightly packed with gauze and a Foley catheter inserted into the bladder.

Broad-ligament haematomas are rare but can occur if a blood vessel ruptures above the pelvic fascia and bleeds between the leaves of the broad ligament. This may extend quite extensively into the retroperitoneal space. The clinical picture will be one of pain and associated hypovolaemia. On bimanual examination, the uterus will be pushed to one side by the broad-ligament mass. Rupture of the uterus should always be considered as a possible cause.

Treatment will involve management of the hypovolaemia with intravenous crystalloid, colloid and blood. If one is sure there is no uterine rupture, the patient is stable and the bleeding is self-limiting, some of these cases can be treated by observation. If, however, there is progression the management may include angiographic embolisation of the branches of the involved internal iliac artery or laparotomy and evacuation of the haematoma. If trauma to the uterus is involved, repair of the rupture or hysterectomy may be required.

UTERINE TAMPONADE

Although packing of the uterus fell into disrepute in the latter part of the 20th century, as it was thought to be ineffective and merely hid the bleeding, it has enjoyed a minor resurgence for specific cases in the 1990s (Maier 1993). To be successful, it requires anaesthesia and tight and systematic packing of the uterine cavity with a gauze roll. The vagina should also be tightly packed and a Foley catheter placed in the bladder. There have been reports of successful uterine tamponade using a Sengstaken–Blakemore tube. The tip of the catheter part of the tube is cut off close to the stomach balloon portion, which is placed in the uterine cavity and inflated with 300 ml of physiological saline (Katsmark *et al.* 1994), while others have used the oesophageal balloon portion inflated with 100–120 ml of physiological saline (Chan *et al.* 1997). A urological hydrostatic balloon catheter has been used for similar effect (Johanson *et al.* 2001). This is kept in place for 12–24 hours and then gradually deflated over several hours and removed. Intrauterine tamponade is best covered with prophylactic antibiotics and a continuous infusion of oxytocin to promote uterine contractions.

MAJOR VESSEL EMBOLISATION

Angiographic embolisation of branches of the internal iliac artery has been used successfully to control haemorrhage from uterine atony as well as trauma to the cervix, paracolpos and upper vagina (Vedanthan *et al.* 1997; Baskett 1999a). Some of the measures mentioned above may be required to sustain the patient until this can be organised. It can be done under local anaesthesia together with mild sedation. Under angiographic control and through a femoral artery puncture, a catheter is guided to the aortic bifurcation and then in turn to each of the internal iliac arteries and its branches. Bleeding vessels are identified by extravasation of contrast material and blocked by the injection of absorbable gelatin (Gelfoam®, Pharmacia) particles.

MAJOR VESSEL LIGATION

If the abdomen is open and one is dealing directly with haemorrhage following caesarean section or uterine rupture, major vessel ligation may be indicated. The most logical approach for uterine haemorrhage is a combination of uterine artery and ovarian artery ligation. Luckily this is simple and can be performed rapidly by any general obstetrician (Figure 16.2) (O'Leary 1974; Fahmy 1987). The placement of the suture, which ligates the ascending branch of the uterine artery, is approximately 2 cm below the level of a transverse lower segment caesarean section incision. Using a large curved needle and a No. 1 USP absorbable suture, pass the needle through the myometrium from front to back, about 2 cm in from the side of the uterus. Transilluminate the broad ligament and bring the needle back through an avascular portion to encircle the uterine vessels. Tie the suture firmly to compress the uterine vessels; this is facilitated and stabilised by the portion of myometrium included in the stitch. Before passing the suture ensure that the bladder is well down to avoid injury to the lower urinary tract. The procedure is repeated on the opposite side. Branches of the ovarian artery pass above the ovary and then down to anastomose with the branches of the ascending uterine artery just below the uterine attachment of the utero-ovarian ligament. An encircling suture is placed just below the utero-ovarian ligament in an identical manner to that used for the uterine artery below. Repeat on the other side. Ligating the ovarian artery at this point does not interfere with the blood supply to the ovary or tube. The uterine arteries usually recanalise

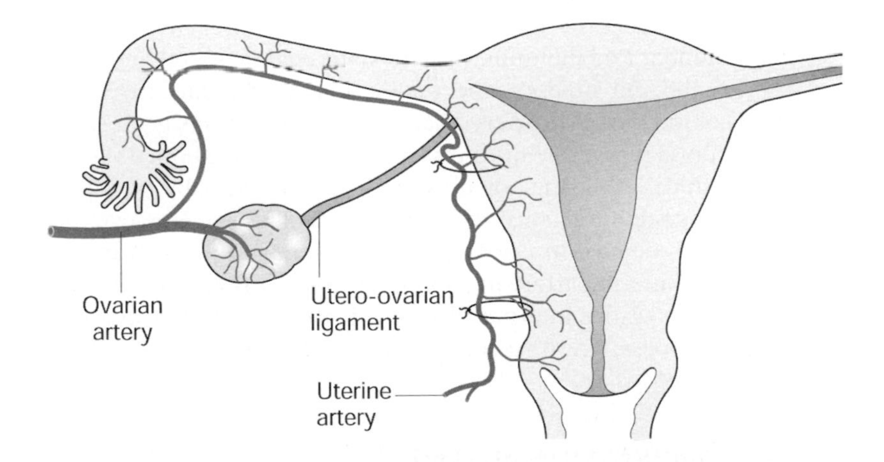

Figure 16.2 Sites for uterine and ovarian artery ligation

and subsequent menstrual and reproductive function is normal. Bilateral uterine and ovarian artery ligation can be achieved swiftly and safely and is often effective in dealing with uterine haemorrhage due to trauma or atony (Abdrabbo 1994).

Internal iliac artery ligation may be considered for haemorrhage from the cervix, paracolpos and upper vagina. Unless the abdomen is already open, it is better to approach these cases with direct suture by the vaginal route and, if this fails, move on to major vessel embolisation. However, if the abdomen is already open or if facilities for vessel embolisation are not available, it is logical to try to deal with the haemorrhage directly. The descending branch of the uterine artery supplies the cervix, vagina and paracolpos. Thus, haemorrhage from these areas is more logically approached by internal iliac artery ligation. The technique is to raise the mid portion of the round ligament with a Babcock clamp and enter the retroperitoneal space between this portion of the round ligament and the fallopian tube. With a finger or sponge stick the space is easily opened to the pelvic sidewall. The bifurcation of the common iliac artery can be seen or palpated. The ureter and its attached peritoneum are adjacent to this bifurcation and must be identified and reflected medially. The external iliac artery passes lateral and superior, with the internal iliac artery passing downwards and medially. Gently clear the areola tissue from the first 3 cm of the internal iliac branch. The artery can then be elevated very gently with a Babcock clamp and a right-angle clamp containing a doubled non-absorbable No. 1 USP suture passed from lateral to medial beneath the artery. This should be done 2–3 cm from the origin of the internal iliac artery and great care must be taken not to damage the adjacent veins underneath the artery. The artery is then doubly ligated but not divided.

Due to the presence of major collateral anastomoses in the pelvis between the lumbar and iliolumbar arteries, the middle sacral and lateral sacral arteries and the superior and middle haemorrhoidal arteries, the effectiveness of internal iliac artery ligation is limited. It has been shown to reduce the pulse pressure within the arterial system by about 85% and, in essence, reduces it to that of a venous system, thereby giving the normal clotting system a chance to work (Burchell 1968). However, it is only about 40% effective in controlling haemorrhage in which medical management and uterine artery ligation have failed. Another drawback is that, with ligation of the internal iliac artery, the access for subsequent angiographic embolisation of vessels is restricted (Clark *et al.* 1985; Evans and McShane 1985).

UTERINE COMPRESSION SUTURE

A number of compression sutures have been devised to stop uterine haemorrhage in an attempt to conserve the uterus. The first of these was described by B-Lynch *et al.* (1997) in five cases. This involved the use of a No. 2 USP absorbable suture and required that the lower uterine segment was opened, as for caesarean section (Figure 16.3). Others have successfully used the same technique and have suggested that, if the uterus was not already opened, the compression suture could be applied without having to make a uterine incision (Ferguson *et al.* 2000; Baskett and Smith 2002; Hayman *et al.* 2002).

Another method is that of multiple square sutures involving a No. 1 USP absorbable suture with four points of entry and exit through the full thickness of the anterior and posterior uterine walls encompassing an approximate 3 cm square (Cho *et al.* 2000). This can be done at multiple sites for uterine atony and may be particularly useful in the lower uterine segment with cases of placenta praevia and/or accreta.

HYSTERECTOMY

All of the above measures are aimed to try to preserve the uterus. Obviously there comes a time in the face of continued and unrelenting haemorrhage when one has to accept the failure of other measures and move to hysterectomy. This will be influenced by the patient's age, parity and desire for future children. The technical aspects of obstetric hysterectomy are covered in Chapter 12.

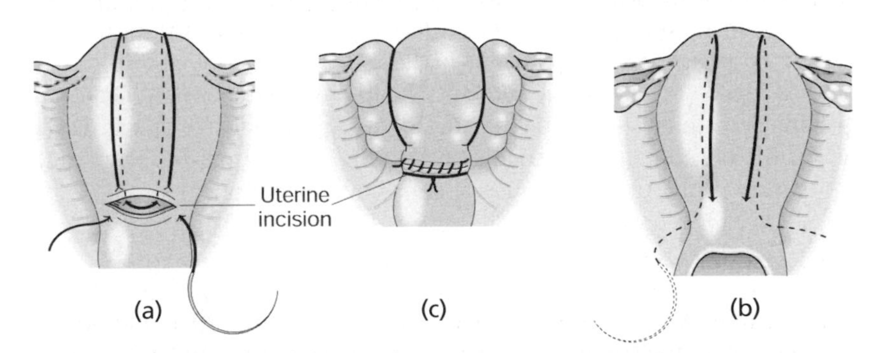

Figure 16.3 Parts (a) and (b) demonstrate the anterior and posterior views of the uterus showing the application of the B-Lynch Brace suture; part (c) shows the anatomical appearance after complete application (original illustration by Mr. Philip Wilson FMAA AIMI, based on the authors' video record of the operation; reproduced with permission from *Br J Obstet Gynaecol* 1997;104:374)

Acute uterine inversion

The frequency of this rare condition depends upon the standard of management of the third stage of labour. The incidence therefore varies widely from one in 2000 to one in 50 000 deliveries. The degree of inversion may be incomplete, in which the fundus is inverted but does not protrude through the cervix, or complete, when the inverted fundus passes completely through the cervix and lies either in the vagina or outside the introitus.

CAUSE

The cause in the majority of cases is mismanagement of the third stage, either by pressure on the uterine fundus or premature traction on the cord before the placenta has separated and when the uterus is relaxed. Less commonly, the condition can occur with a sudden and violent rise in intra-abdominal pressure from coughing or vomiting with the uterus relaxed. It can also happen with too rapid withdrawal of the placenta during manual removal.

DIAGNOSIS

The diagnosis is usually obvious, with the sudden appearance of a boggy mass in the vagina or at the introitus. This is associated with the sudden onset of profound hypotension, bradycardia and pallor. Initially, the shock is of a neurogenic type due to traction on the infundibulopelvic, round and ovarian ligaments. This is usually rapidly followed by hypovolaemic shock from the concurrent bleeding. Occasionally, if the placenta remains entirely attached, the bleeding will be less. Incomplete inversion may be more difficult to diagnose and is usually associated with persistent bleeding. In a thin patient one may be able to appreciate the dimple in the fundus of the uterus, but usually this is only discovered during manual exploration of the uterus because of continued bleeding.

MANAGEMENT

Even though the initial shock is of the neurogenic type, one should assume that hypovolaemia will soon follow (Wendell and Cox 1995). Therefore, two intravenous lines should be established with wide-bore cannulae and crystalloid rapidly infused. Four units of blood should be crossmatched. The majority of these cases, even in hospitals with readily available anaesthesia, require transfusion.

Soon after inversion, the cervical ring will cause constriction and increasing congestion of the inverted fundus. However, if immediate manual replacement of the uterine fundus is carried out, the cervical ring is occasionally relaxed enough to allow successful reduction. This should be tried at once and without waiting for anaesthesia.

MANUAL REPLACEMENT

If manual replacement cannot be carried out easily, anaesthesia has to be given. This usually requires general anaesthesia and a tocolytic to relax the uterus. During manual replacement, do not remove the placenta if it is still attached to the fundus. Replace the fundus with the attached placenta and, once replaced, carry out manual removal of the placenta. Cupping the whole fundus in your hand, lift the entire uterus up out of the pelvis and towards the umbilicus (Figure 16.4). You may have to sustain this pressure for two to four minutes. Once the inversion has been corrected and the placenta, if still attached, is removed, an oxytocin infusion should be run in to contract the uterus. The uterus is then re-explored to make sure that it is intact and there are no remaining placental fragments. An oxytocin infusion should be continued for 8–12 hours.

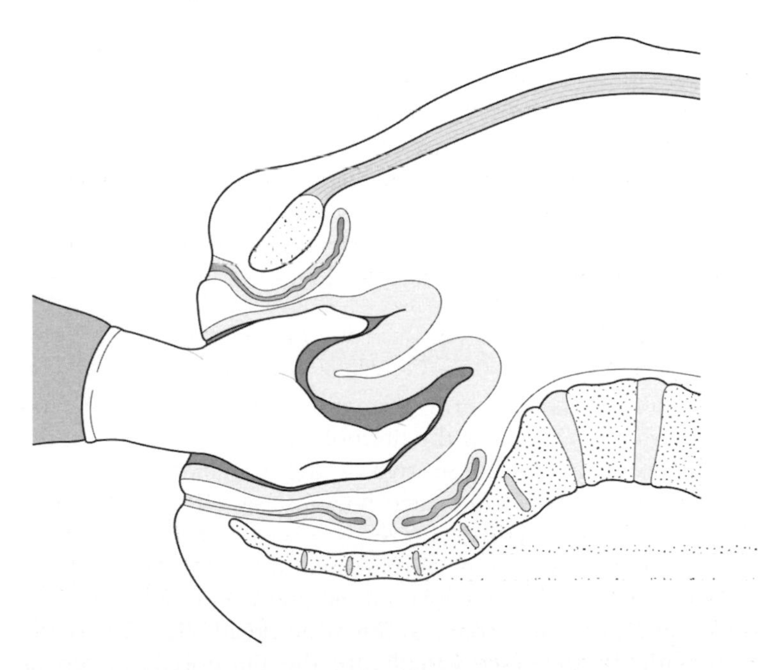

Figure 16.4 Manual replacement of uterine inversion

A tocolytic agent may be required to relax the cervical constriction ring. This is usually best achieved with intravenous glyceryl trinitrate given in doses of 100–200 μg every two to three minutes until there is adequate relaxation. If one is in a situation where general anaesthesia is not feasible, then it may be possible to achieve manual replacement with the use of a tocolytic agent and intravenous morphine.

Provided that anaesthesia is available within one hour of the event it is usually feasible to achieve manual replacement of the uterus under anaesthesia.

If not the hydrostatic method of O'Sullivan may be necessary (O'Sullivan 1945; Mamani and Hassan 1989).

Hydrostatic method of O'Sullivan

The principle of this method is to distend the vaginal fornices with fluid, which pulls outward on the constricting cervical ring in addition to pressure on the inverted uterus, thereby allowing replacement of the inversion. Having ensured that there are no tears in the vagina, cervix or uterus, intravenous tubing is guided into the posterior fornix while the other hand seals the vulva around the forearm. Warm saline is then fed in through the tubing using a pressure infuser; up to five litres may be required.

Huntington's technique and Haultain's operation

In exceptional cases of neglected uterine inversion the above treatments may not succeed. On these rare occasions laparotomy is required to apply Huntington's technique, which involves sequential traction on the inverted fundus with tenacula until it is reduced. Occasionally, at laparotomy the constriction ring is too tight to allow Huntington's technique, in which case Haultain's operation is used with incision of the cervical constriction ring posteriorly. This allows correction of the inversion and the incised portion of the lower uterus is then sutured.

Disseminated intravascular coagulation

Normal coagulation leads to fibrin formation. Once the fibrin has performed its coagulation function the fibrinolytic system disposes of the fibrin. The balance between these two – the coagulation and the fibrinolytic systems – ensures normal haemostasis. In disseminated intravascular coagulation (DIC) there is excess and generalised coagulation due to the release of thromboplastins into the maternal circulation. This causes excessive consumption and eventually depletion of the coagulation factors. Secondary to this widespread coagulation and deposition of fibrin in the microvasculature the fibrinolytic system is activated. The breakdown of fibrin forms fibrin degradation products.

Fibrin degradation products inhibit both thrombin and platelet function, which aggravates the coagulation defect.

In pregnant patients, DIC is always secondary to another initiating condition, which may lead to postpartum haemorrhage. These initiating conditions include placental abruption, amniotic fluid embolism and uterine rupture. They probably initiate DIC by the release of thromboplastins into the maternal circulation from the damaged placental and decidual tissue. In conditions such as severe pre-eclampsia, eclampsia and sepsis, injury to the vascular endothelial cells may expose the underlying collagen and initiate DIC. Hypovolaemic shock and massive blood transfusion may, in their own right, lead to DIC.

CLINICAL PRESENTATION

Clinical presentation is that of the underlying cause, associated with haemorrhagic manifestations such as profuse bleeding from operative sites and the postpartum uterus, together with more subtle signs such as bruising, purpura and constant oozing from venepuncture sites. In addition, extensive DIC may be associated with widespread microvascular thrombosis, which can lead to organ ischaemia and infarction. These later manifestations are usually renal, hepatic or pulmonary dysfunction.

DIAGNOSIS

The diagnosis is usually made on the above clinical features, allied to a variety of haematological tests. It is emphasised, however, that the process of DIC is so dynamic that the interpretation of test results can be difficult as they constantly change and, when received, may not reflect the current haematological state of the patient. When possible, consultation with a haematologist is desirable in these cases. The following tests may be of assistance:

- Both the prothrombin time and thrombin time are usually prolonged.
- The partial thromboplastin time may be normal early in the process and only become prolonged late when the coagulation factors are severely depleted.
- Platelet levels usually fall progressively.
- The serum fibrinogen level is usually increased in pregnancy to 400–640 mg/dl. The level falls with DIC but may remain in the normal non-pregnant range. In severe DIC it will usually fall below 150 mg/dl.
- Fibrinogen and fibrin degradation products are produced with DIC: levels above 80 mg/dl confirm the diagnosis. Even after the process of DIC has been controlled these levels may remain elevated for 24–48 hours.

- As red blood cells are forced through the fibrin mesh in the microvasculature they become abnormally shaped and fragmented. A blood smear may show these abnormally shaped 'schistocytes'.
- If there is widespread destruction of red cells, microangiopathic haemolytic anaemia will ensue resulting in haemolysis and haemoglobinuria.

MANAGEMENT

DIC can develop and progress rapidly. The mainstay of management is to treat the initiating obstetric cause. Once this has been controlled and while this treatment is underway, the patient's circulation must be restored and maintained, together with replacement of procoagulants (Clark *et al.* 1997; ACOG 1998; Baskett 1999b).

The principles of maintaining the circulation and organ perfusion include:

- Rapid infusion of crystalloid, colloid and packed red cells. Fresh whole blood with its full complement of procoagulants is best but this is almost never available.
- Oxygen by facemask. Endotracheal intubation and ventilation may be required.
- If facilities are available, monitor the circulation with a central venous pressure line. If not, try and keep the haematocrit greater than 30% and the urinary output more than 30 ml/hour.
- The replacement of procoagulants should be guided by a haematologist if available. As the initiating cause of the DIC is removed, it is logical to sustain the patient with the addition of procoagulants to maintain haemostasis.
- Fresh frozen plasma contains all the clotting factors. The guiding principle is to give one unit of fresh frozen plasma after the initial transfusion of five units of blood. Thereafter, one unit of fresh frozen plasma is given for every two units of packed red cells transfused.
- Cryoprecipitate is rich in fibrinogen, Von Willebrand factor and factors 8 and 13. It is given for severe hypofibrinogenaemia.
- Severe thrombocytopenia may require platelet transfusion. Each unit of platelets will raise the count by approximately 5000–10 000/ml.
- Under the guidance of a haematologist antithrombin III concentrate may be required.
- Recently, recombinant activated factor 7a has become available and significantly reduces the prothrombin time and partial thromboplastin time. Clotting is activated at the site of the bleeding as local tissue factor

is needed for factor 7a to function (White *et al.* 1999). Studies are required to delineate a potential role in obstetric haemorrhage.

In obstetrics, the vast majority of these patients are young healthy women and, provided that the initiating cause is removed and their circulation and organ perfusion maintained during the crisis, they will recover completely.

References

Abdrabbo SA. (1994) Step-wise uterine devascularization: a novel technique for management of uncontrolled postpartum hemorrhage with preservation of the uterus. *Am J Obstet Gynecol* 171;694–700.

ACOG. (1998) *Postpartum Hemorrhage. Education Bulletin No. 243.* Washington DC: American College of Obstetricians and Gynecologists.

B-Lynch C, Coker A, Lowell AH, Abu J, Cowan MJ. (1997) The B-Lynch surgical technique for the control of massive postpartum haemorrhage: an alternative to hysterectomy? Five cases reported. *Br J Obstet Gynaecol* 104:372–5.

Baskett TF. (1999a) Obstetric haemorrhage: major vessel ligation and embolisation. In: *Essential Management of Obstetric Emergencies.* 3rd ed. Bristol: Clinical Press. p. 242–8.

Baskett TF. (1999b) Disseminated intravascular haemorrhage in pregnancy. In: *Essential Management of Obstetric Emergencies.* 3rd ed. Bristol: Clinical Press. p. 87–92.

Baskett TF, Smith KL. (2002) Uterine compression sutures for severe postpartum haemorrhage. *Obstet Gynecol* 99:76S.

Burchell RC. (1968) Physiology of internal iliac artery ligation. *J Obstet Gynaecol Br Cwlth* 75:642–51.

Chan C, Razyi K, Tham KF, Arulkumaran S. (1997) The use of a Sengstaken–Blakemore tube to control postpartum haemorrhage. *Int J Gynaecol Obstet* 58:251–2.

Cho JH, Jun HS, Lee CN. (2000) Hemostatic suturing technique for uterine bleeding during cesarean delivery. *Obstet Gynecol* 96:129–31.

Clark SL, Phelan JP, Bruce SR, Paul RH. (1985) Hypogastric artery ligation for obstetric hemorrhage. *Obstet Gynecol* 66:353–6.

Clark SL, Cotton DB, Hankins GAV, Phelan JP, editors. (1997) Disseminated intravascular coagulation. In: *Critical Care Obstetrics.* 3rd ed. Oxford: Blackwell Science. p. 551–63.

Evans S, McShane P. (1985) The efficacy of internal iliac ligation. *Surg Gynecol Obstet* 162:250–3.

Fahmy K. Uterine artery ligation to control postpartum haemorrhage. *Int J Gynaecol Obstet* 25:363–7.

Ferguson JE, Bourgeois J, Underwood PB. (2000) B-Lynch suture for postpartum hemorrhage. *Obstet Gynecol* 95:1020–2.

Hayman RG, Arulkumaran S, Steer PJ. (2002) Uterine compression sutures: surgical management of postpartum hemorrhage. *Obstet Gynecol* 99: 502–6.

Johanson R, Kumar M, Obhrai M, Young P. (2001) Management of massive postpartum haemorrhage: use of hydrostatic balloon catheter to avoid laparotomy. *Br J Obstet Gynaecol* 108:420–2.

Katsmark M, Brown R, Raju KS. (1994) Successful use of a Sengstaken–Blakemore tube to control massive postpartum haemorrhage. *Br J Obstet Gynaecol* 101:259–60.

Maier RC. (1993) Control of postpartum hemorrhage with uterine packing. *Am J Obstet Gynecol* 169:17–23.

Mamani AW, Hassan A. (1989) Treatment of puerperal uterine inversion by the hydrostatic method. Report of five cases. *Eur J Obstet Gynecol Reprod Biol* 32:281–5.

O'Brien P, El-Refaey H, Gordon A, Geary M, Rodeck CH. (1998) Rectally administered misoprostol for the treatment of postpartum hemorrhage unresponsive to oxytocin and ergometrine: a descriptive study. *Obstet Gynecol* 92:212–14.

O'Leary JA. (1974) Uterine artery ligation for control of postpartum hemorrhage. *Obstet Gynecol* 43:849–53.

O'Sullivan JV. (1945) Acute inversion of the uterus. *BMJ* ii:282–4.

Tamizian O, Arulkumaran S. (2000) The surgical management of postpartum haemorrhage. *Curr Opin Obstet Gynecol* 13:127–31.

Vedanthan S, Goodwin SC, McLucas B, Mohr G. (1997) Uterine artery embolization: an underused method of controlling pelvic hemorrhage. *Am J Obstet Gynecol* 176:938–48.

Wendell PJ, Cox SM. (1995) Emergent obstetric management of uterine inversion. *Obstet Gynecol Clin North Am* 22:261–74.

White B, McHale J, Ravi N, Reynolds J, Stephens R, Moriarty J, *et al.* (1999) Successful use of recombinant factor VIIa (Novo seven) in the management of intractable post-surgical intra-abdominal haemorrhage. *Br J Haematol* 107: 677–8.

17 Amniotic fluid embolism

A rare event, one in 50 000–100 000 deliveries, amniotic fluid embolism (AFE) is perhaps the most catastrophic of all obstetric complications. In the developed world it accounts for approximately 10% of all direct maternal deaths and is in the top three such causes (Ratten 1988; Burrows and Khoo 1995; Lewis and Drife 2001). Its prominence is accounted for by the fact that, although rare, mortality is 60–80% and, even in those surviving, the hypoxic insult is so profound that the majority have permanent neurological damage.

Pathophysiology

The pathophysiology of AFE is poorly understood. It has been suggested that many of the hallmarks of AFE are similar to those of septic shock and anaphylaxis (Azegami and Mori 1986; Clark *et al.* 1995; Benson and Lindberg 1996; Khang 1998; Clark 1990). Furthermore, it has been established that amniotic fluid commonly enters the maternal circulation without ill effect in most women (Clark *et al.*1986). It is postulated that in certain susceptible women fetal cells and other vasoactive substances, such as prostaglandins and leukotrienes may initiate, via endogenous mediators, a complex pathophysiological cascade similar to that seen in anaphylactic and septic shock. The sequelae are:

- Initially, acute pulmonary arteriolar obstruction and hypertension. This is transient and soon followed by left ventricular failure resulting in profound hypotension (Girard *et al.* 1986; Clark *et al.* 1988.
- Severe hypoxia due to ventilation-perfusion imbalance. This, together with the profound hypotension, produces a generalised hypoxia often leading to seizures. It is this profound and sustained hypoxia that is responsible for the neurological damage in survivors.
- DIC is an almost universal finding in those who survive longer than one hour. This is probably caused by fetal antigens and tissue factors in the amniotic fluid activating the coagulation cascade (Lockwood *et al.* 1991). The DIC is almost certainly compounded by the continuing hypoxia.

Clinical features

ASSOCIATED FACTORS

Reviews have shown that there are no consistent risk factors for AFE (Burrows and Khoo 1995; Clark *et al.* 1995). It is more likely to happen in late pregnancy but can occur in association with first- and second-trimester abortion. Amniotic fluid may gain entry to the maternal circulation during spontaneous labour and delivery or at the time of amniotomy or caesarean section. There are minor associations with certain factors such as: increasing maternal age, high parity, induction or augmentation of labour, operative delivery and minor procedures such as intrauterine pressure catheter insertion, amnioinfusion and amniotomy (Lau and Chui 1994; Maher *et al.* 1994; Lewis and Drife 2001). Some reviews suggest that uterine hyperstimulation is a potential factor and should be avoided (Weiwen *et al.* 2000). However, these associations are quite inconsistent and the condition is therefore unpredictable. The majority of cases occur during labour or just after delivery. On rare occasions, the acute manifestations of AFE may be delayed for two to four hours following delivery (Margarson 1995).

CLINICAL PRESENTATION

Clinical signs and symptoms of AFE include most or all of the following:

- acute respiratory distress, chest discomfort, and cyanosis
- profound hypotension and cardiovascular collapse
- severe hypoxia with loss of consciousness, seizures and/or coma
- haemorrhage and DIC develop in almost all cases if the patient survives for one to two hours.

If the fetus has not been delivered, the maternal hypoxia will soon result in fetal hypoxia manifested by fetal heart rate abnormalities. On occasions there may be tetanic uterine contractions in the early phase following amniotic fluid embolism.

DIAGNOSIS

The differential diagnosis includes other acute events such as pulmonary acid aspiration, thrombotic pulmonary embolism, eclampsia and anaphylactic drug reaction. In most cases, clinical features should distinguish these conditions.

In essence, the sudden onset of cardio-pulmonary collapse, together with coma or seizures, in labour at or shortly after delivery in the woman with no other apparent predisposing causes, should prompt the diagnosis of AFE.

The definitive diagnosis is said to be confirmed by the presence of amniotic fluid debris in the maternal circulation. This can be demonstrated at postmortem examination in the pulmonary precapillary arterioles, with special fat stains and immunohistochemical techniques to identify fetal iso-antigens (Kobayashi *et al.* 1997). In survivors, blood to test for fetal squamous cells may be obtained from the right side of the heart via a central line. However, it has been shown that this may occur in normal pregnancy (Clark *et al.* 1986). Thus, the diagnosis is now largely based on the combination of a clear clinical picture, postmortem analysis, and newer immunohistochemical techniques (Kobayashi *et al.* 1997; Benson *et al.* 2001), with the presence of squames in the maternal circulation a more secondary feature.

Management

The principles of management of this condition are those of resuscitation and intensive care:

- Cardiopulmonary resuscitation, which will include intubation and oxygenation by intermittent positive pressure ventilation.
- Circulatory support with intravenous dopamine infusion may help maintain adequate cardiac output. This is best guided by experts, together with more sophisticated monitoring including central venous pressure, systemic and pulmonary arterial lines.
- Although there is no proof of their value, many will use high-dose steroids such as intravenous hydrocortisone 500 mg every six hours.
- If the patient survives long enough, DIC will almost certainly ensue and the principles of managing this are outlined in Chapter 16.
- If the fetus has not already been delivered, steps should be taken to do so immediately – vaginally if safe and feasible, if not, then by immediate caesarean section. Not only will the fetus rapidly become hypoxic and need to be delivered but resuscitation of the mother will be aided by delivery of the fetus (Greene 1998; Gilbert and Danielsen 1999). Unfortunately, the incidence of neurological damage in both maternal and neonatal survivors is high in this devastating condition.

AFE is so rare that most obstetricians will never encounter a case in their career. National registries have been established in an attempt to gather enough cases to provide insight into this enigmatic and unpredictable condition (Clark *et al.* 1995; Lewis and Drife 2001).

References

Azegami M, Mori N. (1986) Amniotic fluid embolism and leukotrienes. *Am J Obstet*

Gynecol 155:1119–23.

Benson MD, Lindberg RE. (1996) Amniotic fluid embolism, anaphylaxis, and tryptase. *Am J Obstet Gynecol* 175:737.

Benson MD, Kobayashi H, Silver RK, Oi H, Greenberger PA, Terao T. (2001) Immunologic studies in presumed amniotic fluid embolism. *Obstet Gynecol* 97:510–14.

Burrows A, Khoo SK. (1995) The amniotic fluid embolism syndrome: 10 years' experience at a major teaching hospital. *Aust N Z J Obstet Gynaecol* 35:245–50.

Clark SL. (1990) New concepts of amniotic fluid embolism: a review. *Obstet Gynecol Surv* 45:360–8.

Clark SL, Pavlova Z, Greenspoon J, Horenstein J, Phelan JP. (1986) Squamous cells in the maternal pulmonary circulation. *Am J Obstet Gynecol* 154:104–6.

Clark SL, Cotton DB, Gonik B, Greenspoon J, Phelan JP. (1988) Central hemodynamic alterations in amniotic fluid embolism. *Am J Obstet Gynecol* 158:1124–6.

Clark SL, Hawkins GDV, Dudley DA, Dildy GA, Porter TF. (1995) Amniotic fluid embolism: analysis of the national registry. *Am J Obstet Gynecol* 172:1158–69.

Gilbert WM, Danielsen B. (1999) Amniotic fluid embolism: decreased mortality in a population-based study. *Obstet Gynecol* 93:973–7.

Girard P, Mal H, Laine J. (1986) Left heart failure in amniotic fluid embolism. *Anesthesiology* 64:262–5.

Greene MF. (1998) Case records of the Massachusetts General Hospital: Amniotic fluid embolism. *N Engl J Med* 338:821–6.

Khang TY. (1998) Expression of endothelin-1 in amniotic fluid embolism and possible pathophysiological mechanism. *Br J Obstet Gynaecol* 105:802–4.

Kobayashi H, Ooi H, Hayakawa H, Arai T, Matsuda Y, Gotoh K, *et al.* (1997) Histological diagnosis of amniotic fluid embolism by monoclonal antibody TKH-2 that recognizes Neu ac α 2-6 Gal Nac epitope. *Hum Pathol* 28:428–33.

Lau G, Chui PP. (1994) Amniotic fluid embolism, a review of ten fatal cases. *Singapore Med J* 35:180–3.

Lewis G, Drife J, editors. *Why Mothers Die 1997–1999. The Fifth Report of the Confidential Enquires into Maternal Deaths in the United Kingdom*. London: RCOG Press.

Lockwood CJ, Bach R, Guha A, Zhou X, Miller WA, Nemerson Y. (1991) Amniotic fluid contains tissue factor, a potent initiator of coagulation. *Am J Obstet Gynecol* 165:1335–41.

Maher JE, Wenstrom KD, Hauth JC, Meis PJ. (1994) Amniotic fluid embolism after saline amnioinfusion: two cases and review of the literature. *Obstet Gynecol* 83:851–4.

Margarson MP. (1995) Delayed amniotic fluid embolism following caesarean section under spinal anaesthesia. *Anaesthesia* 50:804–6.

Ratten GJ. (1988) Amniotic fluid embolism-two case reports and a review of maternal deaths from this cause in Australia. *Aust N Z J Obstet Gynaecol* 28:33–5.

Weiwen Y, Niugyu Z, Lauxiang Z, Yu L. (2000) Study of the diagnosis and management of amniotic fluid embolism: 38 cases of analysis. *Obstet Gynecol* 95(4 Suppl):38S.

18 Severe pre-eclampsia and eclampsia

Hypertensive disease in pregnancy is a major cause of maternal and perinatal death and morbidity in both developed and developing countries. Severe pre-eclampsia and eclampsia is a multi-organ disease process of undetermined aetiology. The definition of severe pre-eclampsia varies but is generally taken to be sustained hypertension greater than 160/100 mmHg, with proteinuria greater than one gram per litre. The addition of convulsions defines eclampsia. In most cases, when severe pre-eclampsia develops termination of the pregnancy is indicated. Conservative management may be considered in carefully selected cases between 25 and 32 weeks of gestation, in order to gain more time for fetal maturity (Odendaal *et al.* 1990; Hall *et al.* 2000). This chapter is concerned with management during labour or when the decision has been taken to terminate the pregnancy by induction of labour or caesarean section.

Clinical and pathological features

There are certain women who are at increased risk of developing pre-eclampsia.

PREDISPOSING FACTORS FOR PRE-ECLAMPSIA

- Family history
- Primigravida
- Age less than 20 years and over 35 years
- Chronic hypertension or renal disease
- Diabetes mellitus
- Multiple pregnancy
- Gestational trophoblastic disease
- Antiphospholipid syndrome

The clinical manifestations depend on the predominant end-organ involvement and effect.

CLINICAL FEATURES OF SEVERE PRE-ECLAMPSIA

- Sustained hypertension > 160/100 mmHg
- Proteinuria > 1g/litre (2 + dipstick)
- ± oedema

ADDITIONAL FEATURES

- Neurological
  - double or blurred vision
  - scotoma
  - frontal headache
  - hyperreflexia and sustained clonus (≥ 3 beats)
- Oliguria
- Epigastric and right hypochondrial pain
- Nausea and vomiting
- Thrombocytopenia
- Abnormal liver function tests
- Pulmonary oedema

HYPERTENSION AND PROTEINURIA

The common underlying pathology in pre-eclampsia is vascular spasm resulting in hypertension. In severe pre-eclampsia the blood pressure exceeds 160/100 mmHg, although the degree of rise of blood pressure is also important. The young primigravid woman whose normal blood pressure is 90/60 mmHg may develop eclampsia with a blood pressure of less than 160/100 mmHg.

Renal involvement is manifest by glomerular endotheliosis in which the capillary endothelial cells are swollen, leading to glomerular ischaemia and reduced glomerular filtration. This leads to oliguria and proteinuria. In severe pre-eclampsia the degree of proteinuria is at least one gram per litre and often greater than five grams in 24 hours.

The classical triad of pre-eclampsia is hypertension, proteinuria and oedema. However, in many cases oedema is absent or minimal. When it is present it is usually most marked in the face and hands. Occult fluid retention is often shown by marked weight gain in the days or weeks before the development of severe pre-eclampsia.

CONVULSIONS

This is the most dramatic manifestation and moves the diagnosis from severe pre-eclampsia to eclampsia, worsening the prognosis for both mother and fetus. The incidence varies from as much as one in 100 in some developing countries to one in 2000–5000 in developed countries (Moller and Lindmark 1986; Softlas *et al.* 1990; Paruk and Moodley 2000). About 40% of cases of eclampsia are antepartum, 20% intrapartum and 40% postpartum. The seizure is of the grand mal type and it is thought to be caused by vasospasm of the cerebral arteries leading to ischaemia and cerebral oedema. Convulsions may be followed by coma, cortical blindness and focal motor deficits. In most cases these are transient. Cerebrovascular haemorrhage complicates 1–2% of cases (Douglas and Redman 1994).

Prodromal symptoms of eclampsia in the severe pre-eclamptic patient include double or blurred vision, scotoma and frontal headache. Many patient are also hyperreflexic but this is too common a finding in women with pre-eclampsia to be a sensitive predictor of eclampsia.

HEPATIC INVOLVEMENT

Vasospasm in the vascular bed of the liver may be associated with intravascular fibrin deposition and periportal haemorrhagic necrosis. Liver enzymes are elevated and, on rare occasions, bleeding can occur beneath the liver capsule and rupture into the peritoneal cavity with catastrophic results.

PULMONARY OEDEMA

This occurs in less than 5% of cases of severe pre-eclampsia and is due to a combination of factors including low colloid osmotic pressure, pulmonary capillary leak, left ventricular dysfunction and iatrogenic fluid overload.

HAEMATOLOGICAL INVOLVEMENT

The hypercoagulable state of all pregnant women is accentuated in pre-eclampsia. This may be due to vasospasm in the vasa vasorum leading to hypoxia and damage of the endothelial walls in the microvasculature. Thus, a low level of DIC may occur, with the most common manifestation being thrombocytopenia (see Chapter 16). Mild thrombocytopenia (< 100 000/ml) is not uncommon but the full picture of microangiopathic haemolytic anaemia or DIC is rare.

HELLP SYNDROME

Within the clinical spectrum of severe pre-eclampsia/eclampsia is the HELLP syndrome (haemolysis, elevated liver enzymes and low platelets). This was first described by Wienstein (1982) and complicates 4–12% of patients with severe pre-eclampsia/eclampsia (Duckett *et al.* 2001). HELLP syndrome may present a wide clinicopathological spectrum, ranging from a gastrointestinal presentation with nausea, vomiting and right upper-quadrant pain, mimicking gall bladder disease and without hypertension, to a florid case with severe pre-eclampsia/eclampsia, jaundice, DIC and severe thrombocytopenia (ACOG 1996).

FETAL EFFECTS

Uteroplacental blood flow, and therefore perfusion to the intervillous space, is often reduced. This may present as fetal intrauterine growth restriction and/or hypoxia. Placental abruption is also more common.

Management

MANAGEMENT OF SEVERE PRE-ECLAMPSIA/ECLAMPSIA

- Protect and maintain airway
- Stop or prevent convulsions
- Treat hypertension/cardiovascular monitoring
- Fluid balance/monitor renal function
- Detection and management of thrombocytopenia and disseminated intravascular coagulation
- Deliver the patient: induction of labour/caesarean section

ANTICONVULSANT THERAPY

Since the Collaborative Eclampsia Trial (Eclampsia Trial Collaborative Group 1995), magnesium sulphate has been established as the treatment of choice for prevention of convulsions (RCOG 1996). Magnesium sulphate prophylaxis should also be applied to patients with severe pre-eclampsia and has been shown to be superior to placebo in randomised trials (Coetzee *et al.* 1998; Magpie Trial Collaborative Group 2002). Each obstetric unit should develop its own guidelines for these cases (RCOG 1996).

Magnesium sulphate acts as a vasodilator and as a membrane stabiliser. It may also have a central anticonvulsant effect (Cotton *et al.* 1992). The initial dose of magnesium sulphate is 4 g by intravenous infusion over 20 minutes. A 50% solution of magnesium sulphate contains one gram per 2 ml. Thus, the loading dose is 8 ml of the 50% solution followed by a maintenance dose of 2 g/hour using a controlled-infusion device (ACOG 1996). High levels of magnesium sulphate can cause fatal respiratory and cardiovascular depression and a careful monitor of continued magnesium sulphate therapy is therefore required. If laboratory facilities are available, biochemical monitoring can be carried out one hour following the initial dose and every four to six hours thereafter. The aim is to keep the magnesium level between two to four mmol/litre (4–8 mg/dl). If laboratory facilities are not available biological monitoring is usually adequate. If the respiratory rate is less than 12/minute, deep tendon reflexes are absent (patella reflex if no epidural, biceps tendon if epidural in place) and oliguria is less than 25 ml/hour, the magnesium sulphate infusion should be stopped and blood levels checked. If laboratory testing is unavailable the magnesium sulphate can be restarted at 1 g/hour when the respiratory rate has come back to normal and the deep tendon reflexes have returned. The presence of oliguria is very important as magnesium sulphate is excreted solely by the kidneys (ACOG 1996).

If magnesium sulphate overdose occurs as shown by the above biological features plus periods of apnoea and deep sedation, the antidote to magnesium sulphate, calcium gluconate 1 g (10 ml of 10% solution) should be given intravenously over two minutes. On rare occasions it may be necessary to support ventilation by mechanical means until the plasma magnesium sulphate levels have fallen.

If the patient is first seen during an eclamptic fit, the fit should be controlled by the bolus dose of magnesium sulphate previously described or with diazepam 10 mg intravenously over one minute. This can be repeated until the seizure abates. This should then be followed by magnesium sulphate prophylaxis as outlined above. Should a patient on magnesium sulphate prophylaxis have a seizure it should be controlled with a bolus dose of magnesium sulphate or diazepam: the plasma level of magnesium sulphate can be checked and the dose adjusted thereafter as required. On rare occasions, the above anticonvulsant therapy is unsuccessful and these patients may require a thiopental drip, muscle relaxants, intubation and assisted ventilation in an intensive care unit.

ANTIHYPERTENSIVE THERAPY

The most serious risk to the mother from the hypertension of pre-eclampsia is cerebral haemorrhage. For this reason, most clinicians advocate hypotensive therapy if the diastolic blood pressure is sustained at greater than 105 mmHg. A balance has to be achieved between this goal and excessive reduction of the blood pressure, which may reduce uteroplacental blood flow and threaten the fetus. The aim is therefore to reduce the blood pressure by 15–20% so that the diastolic is in the 90–100 mmHg range. The most commonly used drug is hydralazine, which is a peripheral vasodilator. The initial dose is 5 mg given intravenously over two minutes. This can be repeated at 15-minute intervals if the blood pressure is not controlled. Intermittent 5 mg intravenous boluses can then be given to maintain the diastolic blood pressure at about 95 mmHg. An alternative is to set up a continuous intravenous infusion at approximately 5 mg/hour and adjust accordingly. Tachycardia and headache, as a result of vasodilatation, are common adverse effects of hydralazine and tachyphylaxis can also occur.

Another suitable hypotensive agent is labetalol, a combined alpha- and beta-adrenergic blocker. It may be used as an alternative to hydralazine or to combat hydralazine-induced tachycardia. The initial dose is 20 mg intravenously; if this is ineffective in 15 minutes, 40 mg should be given intravenously. A continuous infusion is then established at 40 mg/hour and adjusted to maintain the diastolic at about 95 mmHg.

FLUID BALANCE/CARDIOVASCULAR MONITORING

Plasma volume is decreased in severe pre-eclampsia. However, the available intravascular space is filled and these patients do not tolerate haemorrhage or the loss of fluid from diuretic administration. On the other hand, attempts to expand the blood volume with intravenous fluid may overload the circulation. Together with the reduced colloid osmotic pressure associated with hypoalbuminaemia, these patients are vulnerable to pulmonary oedema. If the vasoconstriction is released by hypotensive agents or epidural regional anaesthesia, additional intravenous fluid will be required to fill the expanded intravascular space. The aim, therefore, is to provide intravenous crystalloid, usually as Ringer-Lactate solution, to cover the insensible loss and urinary output. One also has to allow for the need for more intravenous fluid if the intravascular space is expanded by hypotensive drugs or regional anaesthesia. While it may not be necessary in all cases, a central venous pressure line may be of assistance in guiding this fluid management (Young and Johanson 2001). The aim is to keep the central venous pressure value between 4 mmHg and 8 mmHg. An initial intravenous infusion of 100 ml/hour is reasonable. One must remember that the fluids infusing the anticonvulsants and hypotensive medications must be included in this figure. An indwelling Foley catheter is required to monitor the urinary output, which should ideally be greater than 25 ml/hour. It may be necessary to monitor left-ventricular function with a

Swan–Ganz catheter if the hypertension is severe and hard to control, if there is marked oliguria or if pulmonary oedema develops. In these cases, the guidance of those regularly involved with intensive care is required and the assistance of the obstetric anaesthetist is essential.

HAEMATOLOGICAL CONSIDERATIONS

The most common abnormality is thrombocytopenia, which is present if the platelet count is less than 100 000/ml. Spontaneous haemorrhage is unlikely to occur unless the level falls below 20 000/ml. However, if caesarean section is required, platelet transfusion may be necessary to keep the count greater than 50 000/ml. If thrombocytopenia develops, the other criteria of the HELLP syndrome should be sought. The rare development of DIC requires the management outlined in Chapter 16.

ANALGESIA AND ANAESTHESIA

If available, epidural analgesia is desirable for pain relief in labour and for operative vaginal or caesarean delivery. The absence of pain, and its associated catecholamine rise, helps control the blood pressure. Greater control of maternal bearing-down effort is also desirable to minimise hypertension. For the reasons mentioned before, epidural anaesthesia will increase the intravascular space and may be associated with acute hypotension unless appropriate pre-loading with intravenous crystalloid is carried out.

General anaesthesia may be required if there is a coagulopathy but this carries increased risks in the presence of laryngeal oedema making intubation difficult or even impossible, as well as the potential to worsen laryngeal oedema and cause postoperative respiratory obstruction. In addition, during induction and recovery from anaesthesia and intubation there is a transient exacerbation of hypertension.

CLINICAL/NURSING CARE

These cases require intensive nursing care and the close supervision of an experienced obstetric consultant. An obstetric anaesthetist should be involved early on during induction and/or labour. Depending upon the complexity of the case and the type of complications, the assistance of other consultants, such as internal medicine, haematology and renal medicine, may be necessary.

The patient should be nursed in a single quiet room with a mouth gag readily available at the bedside to place between the jaws and protect the tongue should an eclamptic convulsion occur.

During the initial loading dose of antihypertensive medication, the blood pressure should be recorded every five minutes. Thereafter it can be taken every 15–30 minutes as the pressure stabilises. The patient's reflexes, respiratory rate, fluid balance and urinary output should be recorded hourly. If applicable, central venous pressure and oxygen saturation should also be recorded hourly.

Delivery

The only cure for severe pre-eclampsia and eclampsia is delivery of the fetus and placenta. The treatment outlined up to now is aimed to protect the mother and fetus until this can be accomplished.

If conditions are favourable for induction of labour then this is the treatment of choice with amniotomy and oxytocin. If the cervix is unfavourable but the maternal and fetal conditions are stable and well controlled, the use of vaginal prostaglandins to induce labour may be acceptable.

Caesarean section is chosen if there are other obstetric indications such as breech presentation, IUGR, fetal compromise or non-progressive labour.

As mentioned above, epidural anaesthesia is the ideal for labour and vaginal delivery. Appropriate use of oxytocin augmentation during the second stage should allow the head to deliver spontaneously with minimal maternal effort or by assisted low pelvis delivery, either by forceps or vacuum. Oxytocin should be used for management of the third stage and ergometrine is specifically contraindicated because of its tendency to precipitate a hypertensive crisis in these patients.

Postpartum considerations

Anticonvulsant therapy should continue for 24 hours. During this time the patient should continue to be treated in an intensive obstetric area with continuous nursing care. Usually, the antihypertensive therapy can be reduced postpartum but occasionally an oral hypotensive agent may be needed for the first two to four weeks postpartum. Thrombocytopenia, if present, tends to reach its nadir 24–30 hours postpartum and then spontaneously recover. A diuresis, which is often quite profound, usually occurs within 12–24 hours.

Severe pre-eclampsia is not common and eclampsia is rare in developed countries. Even large obstetric units may only see up to two eclamptic cases per year. It is necessary for all obstetric units to have guidelines and protocols for management of these cases. Consistent application of these guidelines and early involvement of experienced medical and nursing staff is essential to ensure the best outcome (ACOG 2002; RCOG 1996).

Before the patient is discharged from hospital, the future outlook for herself and subsequent pregnancies should be discussed. She has approximately 10–20% chance of developing pre-eclampsia in another pregnancy. This advice can be fine-tuned depending upon the presence of other factors, such as chronic hypertension, antiphospholipid syndrome, etc.

References

ACOG. (1996) *Hypertension in Pregnancy. Technical Bulletin No. 219*. Washington DC: American College of Obstetricians and Gynecologists.

ACOG. (2002) *Diagnosis and Management of Preeclampsia and Eclampsia. Practice Bulletin No. 33*. Washington DC: American College of Obstetricians and Gynecologists.

Coetzee EJ, Dommisse J, Anthony J. (1998) A randomised controlled trial of intravenous magnesium sulphate versus placebo in the management of women with severe pre-eclampsia. *Br J Obstet Gynaecol* 105:300–3.

Cotton DB, Janusz CA, Berman RF. (1992) Anticonvulsant effects of magnesium sulfate on hippocampal seizures: therapeutic implications in pre-eclampsia/eclampsia. *Am J Obstet Gynecol* 16:1127–36.

Douglas KA, Redman CW. (1994) Eclampsia in the United Kingdom. *BMJ* 309:1395–400.

Duckett RA, Kenny L, Baker PN. (2001) Hypertension in pregnancy. *Curr Obstet Gynaecol* 11:7–14.

Eclampsia Trial Collaborative Group. (1995) Which anticonvulsant for women with eclampsia? Evidence from the Collaborative Eclampsia Trial. *Lancet* 345:1455–63.

Hall DR, Odendaal HJ, Steyn DW, Grové D. (2000) Expectant management of early onset severe pre-eclampsia: maternal outcome. *Br J Obstet Gynaecol* 107:1252–7.

Moller B, Lindmark G. (1986) Eclampsia in Sweden, 1976–80. *Acta Obstet Gynecol Scand* 65:307-14.

Odendaal HJ, Pattinson RC, Bom R, Grové D, Kotze TJ. (190) Aggressive or expectant management for women with severe pre-eclampsia between 28–34 weeks gestation: a randomised controlled trial. *Obstet Gynecol* 76:1070–5.

Paruk F, Moodley J. (2000) Treatment of severe pre-eclampsia/eclampsia syndrome. In: Studd J, editor. *Progress in Obstetrics and Gynaecology Volume 14*. Edinburgh: Churchill Livingstone. p. 102–19.

RCOG. (1996, reviewed 1999) *Management of Eclampsia. Guideline. No. 10*. London: Royal College of Obstetricians and Gynaecologists.

Softlas AF, Olsen DR, Franks AL, Atrash HK, Pokras R. (1990) Epidemiology of pre-eclampsia and eclampsia in the United States 1976–1986. *Am J Obstet Gynecol* 163:460–5.

The Magpie Trial Collaborative Group. (2002) Do women with pre-eclampsia, and their babies, benefit from magnesium sulphate? The Magpie Trial: a randomised placebo-controlled trial. *Lancet* 359:1877–90.

Wienstein L. (1982) Syndrome of hemolysis, elevated liver enzymes and low platelet count: a severe consequence of hypertension in pregnancy. *Am J Obstet Gynecol* 142:159–64.

Young P, Johanson R. (2001) Haemodynamic, invasive and echocardiographic monitoring in the hypertensive parturient. *Clin Obstet Gynaecol* 15:605–22.

19 Neonatal resuscitation

Only 1–2% of neonates will require active resuscitation. Anticipation of deliveries where problems may occur, rapid and accurate assessment of the newborn and application of practical resuscitation techniques are required by all those attending deliveries.

ANTICIPATING PROBLEMS: EXAMPLES WHERE RESUSCITATION MAY BE REQUIRED

- Preterm deliveries less than 35 weeks completed gestation
- Emergency caesarean deliveries
- Breech birth
- Fetal distress
- Thick meconium
- Expected major fetal abnormality
- Concern for other reasons, e.g. maternal drug addiction

Assessment

The condition of the baby at birth is traditionally defined using the Apgar score (Table 19.1). However, most useful in deciding whether the baby needs resuscitation or not is a rapid assessment of breathing, heart rate and colour.

Table 19.1 The Apgar scoring system

Measure score	*0*	*1*	*2*
Heart rate	Absent	< 100 bpm	> 100 bpm
Respiratory effort	Absent	Slow, irregular	Regular with crying
Muscle tone	Limp	Some tone in limbs	Active flexion
Reflex irritability	Nil	Grimace only	Vigorous crying
Colour	Pale	Pink with blue extremities	Pink

RAPID ASSESSMENT

- **Breathing**
  Check rate and quality.
- **Heart rate**
  Listen to the apex beat with a stethoscope, palpate the brachial or femoral pulse or palpate the base of the umbilical cord.
- **Colour**
  Look at the trunk, lips and tongue – note if the baby is centrally pink, cyanosed or pale. Peripheral cyanosis is common and by itself does not indicate hypoxaemia.

After assessing breathing, heart rate and colour, the baby can usually be placed in one of four broad categories:

- healthy
- primary apnoea
- terminal apnoea
- fresh stillbirth.

HEALTHY

- Pink; crying lustily; heart rate greater than 100 bpm.

ACTION: dry and give to mother.

PRIMARY APNOEA

- Cyanosed; heart rate greater than 100 bpm; some respiratory effort, tone and response to stimulation.

ACTION: gentle stimulation and facial oxygen.

This baby is likely to begin to breathe spontaneously; a short wait of not more than one minute is acceptable. Stimulate by rubbing with a dry towel, gentle oral or nasal suction, oxygen to the face. If no response by one minute, use bag-and-mask ventilation.

TERMINAL APNOEA

- Pale; heart rate less than 60 bpm; floppy and apnoeic.

ACTION: bag and mask ventilation immediately.

This baby will not breathe without help; if not improving quickly intubation and cardiac compressions will be required.

FRESH STILLBIRTH

- Apnoeic; pale; floppy; no heart rate.

ACTION: full cardiopulmonary resuscitation immediately (follow A B C set out below).

Assist breathing: positive pressure ventilation via endotracheal tube (or with bag and mask) until skilled help for intubation available. Give cardiac compressions.

The A B C of resuscitation

- **A**irway
- **B**reathing
- **C**irculation

The **A B C** approach, with some additions, is used and the practical aspects are discussed in this section.

- **Temperature control – keep the baby warm**

Keeping the baby dry and warm reduces the risk of hypoglycaemia and acidosis and minimises oxygen consumption. The baby is placed on the resuscitaire and rapidly dried with warm towels. Make sure that the radiant heater is on and the clock started.

- **Assess the baby's condition**

By assessing breathing, heart rate and colour (see above section) it is obvious in most cases whether resuscitation is necessary or not.

Airway

Position the baby face upwards with the head in the neutral position. Use soft suction catheters and a negative pressure of 5–10 kPa to gently clear airway. Avoid deep pharyngeal suction as vagal stimulation can cause bradycardia or laryngospasm. A gentle stream of oxygen can be directed towards the nose and mouth and further stimulation provided by rubbing the baby's body with a towel.

Breathing

After establishing a clear airway assist the breathing if:

- shallow irregular respiration with heart rate less than 100bpm and falling
- apnoea.

Intubation is the most efficient way of ventilating the lungs but should only be attempted by a skilled person. Bag-and-mask ventilation is satisfactory and a necessary skill for all those attending deliveries.

BAG-AND-MASK VENTILATION

Choose a mask big enough to cover the face from the bridge of the nose to below the mouth. Make sure that there is good contact with the face so that an effective seal is created (Figure 19.1). Connect the bag to an oxygen supply. A reservoir should be attached to the bag to maximise oxygen delivery. The bag usually has a blow-off valve that operates at 30–40 cm H_2O. This is usually sufficient to provide an adequate tidal volume and minimises the risk of pneumothorax. Squeeze the bag to achieve adequate chest expansion. As a guide, the lower sternum should lift by 1–2 cm with each squeeze of the bag. Establish a rate of 30–40 breaths per minute.

On some resuscitaires it is also possible to give effective ventilation via a T-piece system connected to the oxygen outlet. Ensure that the pressure blow-off valve on the resuscitaire is set at the correct pressure (25–30 cm H_2O is usually satisfactory). The hole on the connector is occluded with a finger to allow the pressure to build up and ventilation is delivered by releasing and reoccluding the hole on the connector at the desired rate. Look at the baby to ensure chest inflation is adequate.

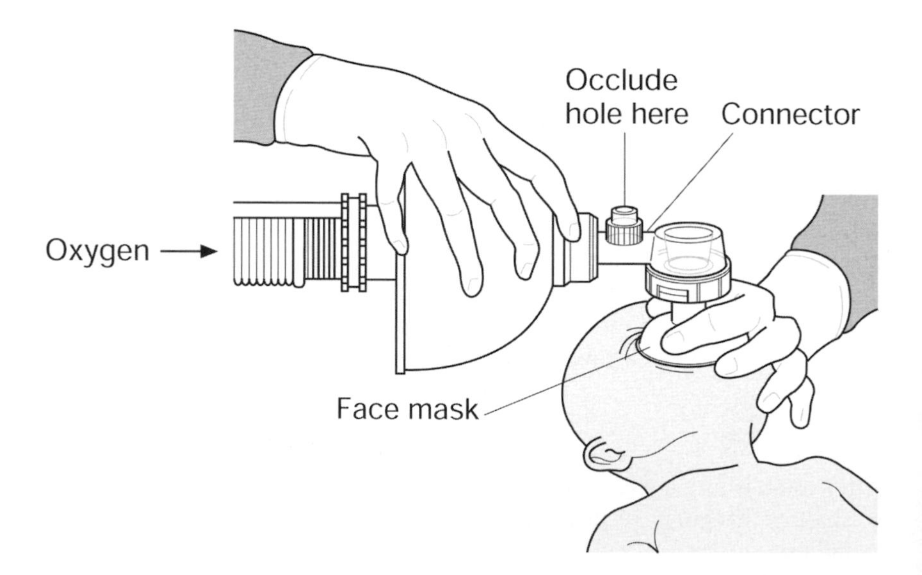

Figure 19.1 Neonatal resuscitation using a bag and mask

INTUBATION

Intubation requires considerable practice. For the skilled person it is indicated if:

- primary apnoea does not respond promptly to bag-and-mask ventilation
- terminal apnoea or asystole.

Figure 19.2 illustrates using the laryngoscope to visualise the structures that allow correct placement of the endotracheal tube. For small babies use size 2.5 mm and for term babies use 3.0–3.5 mm.

Hold the first inflation for two or three seconds to allow proper expansion of the lungs and to establish a functional residual capacity. After the first few breaths, establish a rate of 30–40 breaths per minute with inspiratory times of approximately 0.5–1.0 second. If there is poor chest movement the pressure can be increased sequentially up to 40 cm H_2O.

Following intubation check for:

- bilateral chest movement
- breath sounds bilateral and equal on auscultation
- absence of breath sounds over the stomach.

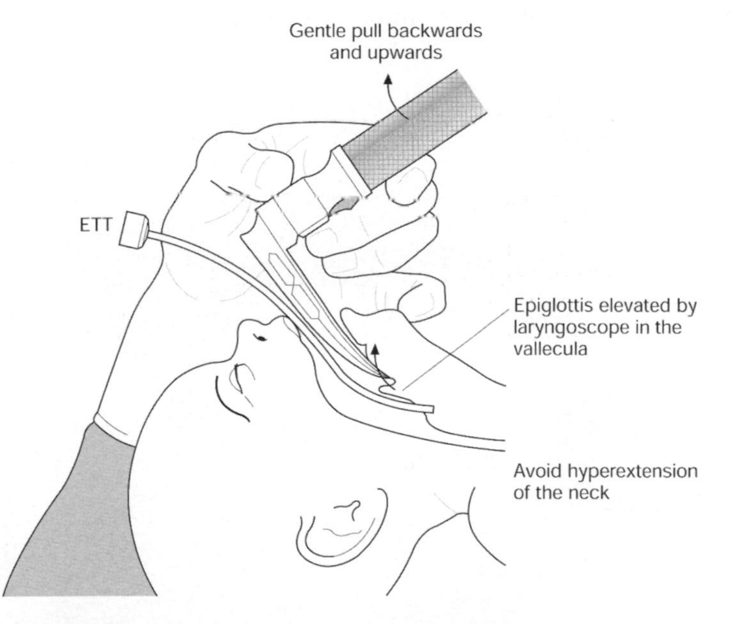

Figure 19.2 Using the laryngoscope to visualise the structures that allow correct placement of the endotracheal tube

Circulation

CARDIAC COMPRESSION

Cardiac compressions are started if the heart rate is less than 60 bpm despite effective ventilation.

This may be performed in one of two ways:

- encircle chest with both hands so that fingers lie behind the baby and thumbs are opposed over the mid-sternum (Figure 19.3). This is the most efficient method.
- place two fingers over the sternum 1 cm below the inter-nipple line (Figure 19.4).

Depress the sternum at a rate of 120 compressions per minute to a depth of 1–2 cm. Give three chest compressions for every inhalation.

DRUGS

Drugs are rarely needed in neonatal resuscitation (Table 19.2). They are indicated if adequate ventilation with 100% oxygen and effective chest compressions have failed to increase the heart rate above 60 bpm.

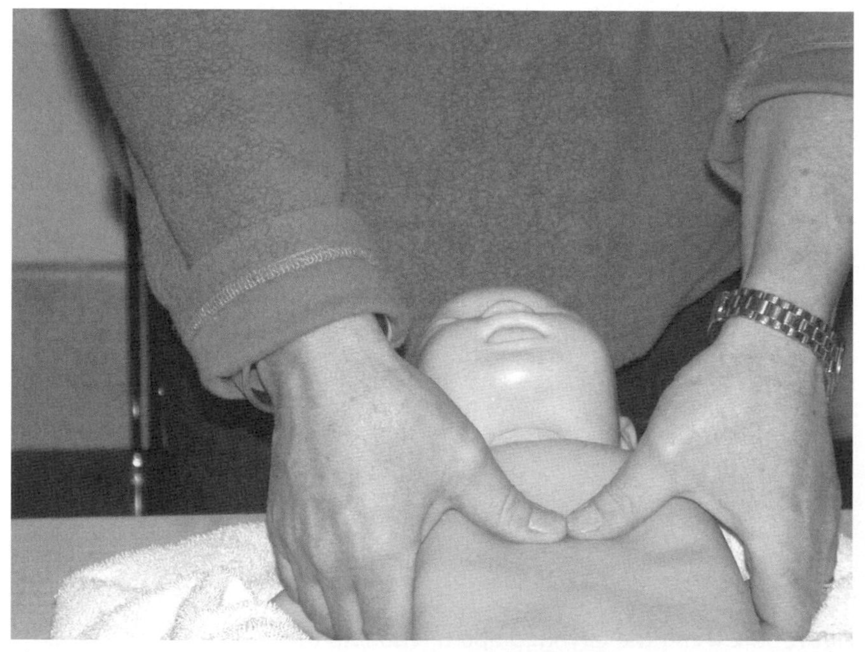

Figure 19.3 Cardiac compression using encircling hands

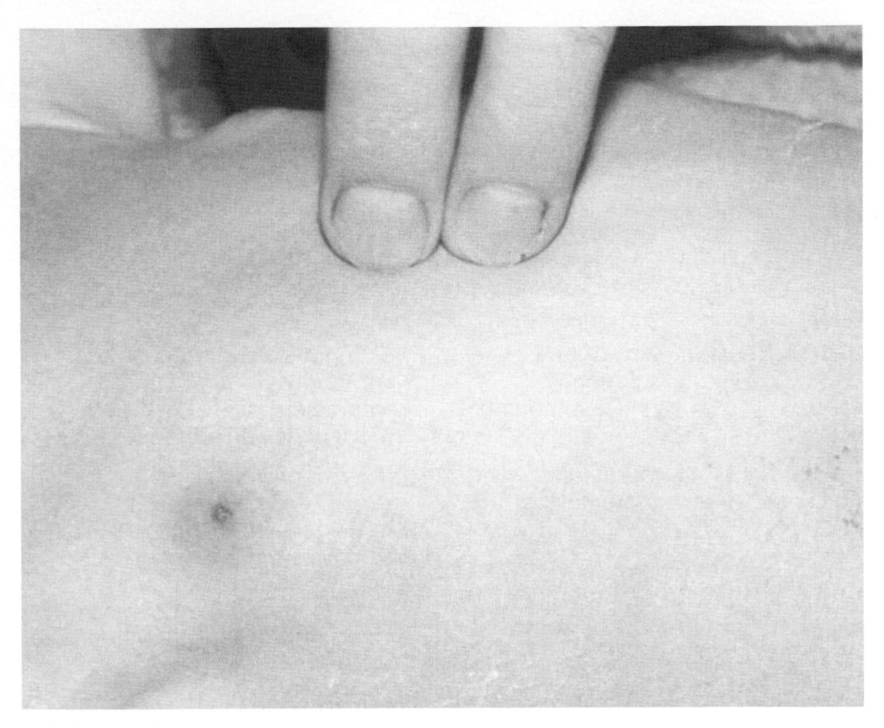

Figure 19.4 Cardiac compression using two fingers

Resuscitation of the infant with meconium stained liquor

When thick meconium is present at delivery, aspirate the mouth and nostrils with a wide-bore suction catheter when the head is delivered. Following delivery, move the baby quickly to the resuscitaire for further assessment.

PINK AND VIGOROUS BABY

If meconium is still present in the oropharynx apply gentle suction. Visualisation of the larynx and intubation are not usually required.

BABY SHOWS DEPRESSION OF RESPIRATORY EFFORT

The pharynx is sucked out before the baby is either encouraged to breathe or given artificial respiratory support. If thick meconium is in the mouth,

Table 19.2 Drugs used in neonatal resuscitation		
Drug	*Dose*	*Indications*
Adrenaline	10 μg/kg (0.1 ml/kg 1 in 10 000) IV **or** 20 μg/kg via endotracheal tube	The most important drug Can be given either intravenously (via umbilical venous catheter) or down the endotracheal tube
	10–30 μg/kg every 3–5 minutes	If no response
Sodium bicarbonate	1 mmol/kg IV: use 2ml/kg of 4.2% solution (= 0.5 mmol/ml)	If the heart rate remains < 60 bpm despite good ventilation, chest compressions and intravenous adrenaline
Volume expanders	10–20 ml/kg over 5–10 minutes	If no response to resuscitation, especially if any evidence of hypovolaemia. Use physiological saline or 4.5% human albumin solution Rhesus negative blood is given when significant acute blood loss is suspected
Dextrose 10%	2–3 ml/kg IV	To avoid hypoglycaemia
Naloxone	100 μg/kg IM	Only for persisting apnoea related to maternal opiate analgesia in an otherwise well baby. It does not improve cardiac performance and should not be given to an asphyxiated baby or a baby whose heart rate is < 60 bpm or if mother is opiate dependent

visualise the larynx and the vocal cords with laryngoscope. Meconium at the level of or below the vocal cords is an indication for intubation and direct suction. Removal of the endotracheal tube and reintubation with a clean tube may be required several times in the presence of thick particulate meconium. This can be continued for up to two minutes in the infant with a good heart rate. Where the heart rate is less than 60 bpm, full resuscitation should be commenced at one minute, even if all the meconium has not been removed.

ACTIONS IN THE EVENT OF POOR INITIAL RESPONSE TO RESUSCITATION

There needs to be constant reassessment of **A B C** during resuscitation. Failure of the baby to improve may indicate a loss of airway patency (e.g. Is the neutral position being maintained? Are there secretions blocking the airway?) or inadequate breathing (e.g. Is there a good mask seal? Is there adequate chest movement?). There should then be a systematic approach to look for other reasons.

FAILURE OF BABY TO IMPROVE: CHECKLIST

1. Check for technical fault.

- Is oxygen connected?
- Is endotracheal tube in the trachea?
- Is endotracheal tube down one bronchus? If in doubt remove tube and replace
- Is endotracheal tube blocked?
- Check blow-off valve set at 30 cm H_2O
- Check flow rate of oxygen at 5–8 litres per minute.

2. Does the baby have lung pathology, e.g.

- pneumothorax
- diaphragmatic hernia
- hypoplastic lungs
- hydrops.

3. If the baby has good chest movement has there been:

- fetal haemorrhage: consider plasma or 0-ve blood 20–30 ml/kg via umbilical vein.
- severe asphyxia.

Resuscitation of the preterm infant

Preterm babies are likely to be deficient in surfactant and may require relative higher inflation pressures than term babies. Start resuscitation with a pressure of 20–25 cm H_2O but increase if this does not produce satisfactory chest wall movement.

When should resuscitation be stopped?

If signs of life were present shortly before delivery it is justifiable to carry out full cardiopulmonary resuscitation on a fresh stillbirth. Published data, however, suggest that if there are still no signs of life by 15 minutes then very few babies will survive. If no response to full resuscitation, the decision to discontinue should be made by the most senior paediatrician available.

Further reading

Advanced Life Support Group. (2000) *Advanced Paediatric Life Support.* 3rd ed. London: BMJ Publishing Group.

American Academy of Pediatrics. (1997) *Paediatric Advanced Life Support.* Elk Grove Village, IL: AAP.

Hamilton, P. (1997) Care of the newborn in the delivery room. *BMJ* 318;1403–6.

Royal College of Paediatrics and Child Health, Royal College of Obstetricians and Gynaecologists. (1997) *Resuscitation of Babies at Birth. A Report of a Joint Working Party of the Royal College of Paediatrics and Child Health and the Royal College of Obstetricians and Gynaecologists.* London: BMJ Publishing Group.

20 Perinatal loss

Families may experience feelings of loss and grief in relation to many aspects of childbearing. This is not just with the obvious experiences of stillbirth and early neonatal death: similar feelings and reactions may occur with miscarriage, infertility, termination, congenital anomaly and adoption. The loss of a baby is something no parent ever forgets – it can cast a 'long shadow' and change the way they see the world. What happens in hospital can have lifelong repercussions on parental grieving. Appropriate professional care and support at this time can be invaluable.

Why is the death of a baby different?

In modern developed society, as death has moved from the home to hospital, death has become more institutionalised. Death is often seen as unfamiliar and frightening, almost a taboo, especially the death of a baby. Birth is seen as a happy, even joyous event and thus death in the birth chamber appears as an obscene contradiction. Many parents may have never experienced death, seen a dead body or even been in a hospital before.

Death may not only be unfamiliar and totally unexpected but also unrehearsed – leading not only to initial shock and confusion but sometimes to quite unexpected reactions.

Feelings and reactions of professionals

Professionals involved may be more familiar with death. However, the death of a baby is often unexpected and can still be painful. We may not have experienced bereavement but we may still experience feelings similar to grief reactions of shock, failure and guilt. It is important to be aware that someone else's grief may also trigger memories and feeling related to our own personal losses. It is natural to turn away from these painful feelings, yet in order to grow and be able to help others it is important to look into ourselves and be willing to recognise that we too need help and support sometimes. Occasionally, after a particularly shocking or traumatic obstetric incident post-traumatic stress may occur and need treatment.

The 'dream' baby

When a woman, her partner and family find out that she is pregnant, they are not expecting an embryo or a fetus but a baby. They may already imagine their son, daughter or grandchild going to school, playing football or going down the aisle. This is the 'dream' baby: this is the baby on television and in magazines. Chubby, with soft downy hair and big eyes, this baby never cries or stays awake all night. When a baby dies all these hopes, plans and dreams for the future die with the baby. This 'dream baby' ideal can also lead to feelings of grief when the baby is not what the parents expected. For example, the birth of a very preterm infant, scrawny with almost transparent skin, or the birth of the 'wrong' sex baby can also lead to feelings of loss.

What a baby means

What a baby means to a woman, couple or family will vary dramatically. For one woman the pregnancy may be unplanned, unwanted and going to turn her life upside down. For another the pregnancy may be a disaster, a nightmare come true, or may have resulted from violence or abuse. Alternatively, a baby may have been planned and prepared for with care, a joy and a fulfilment. This baby may have been the result of years of fertility treatment or a last attempt to save a failing relationship. For every expectant parent, the baby is going to mean something different and unique and the death of that baby will lead to different feelings, reactions and individual needs.

Bereavement and grief

Bereavement is 'the fact of loss' and originally comes from 'to reave' meaning 'to be violently robbed or plundered'. For parents whose baby has died, the connotation of loss or having something precious snatched away are both appropriate. Loss can be a useful word, as it is non-specific, covering many situations, and suggests that the bereaved parents have been passive in the event. However the word 'loss' may also imply carelessness or irresponsibility. This is an example of how important the words we use can be and how sensitive we need to be when using them. For example, to parents the medical term abortion, although correct, may have implications that the more sensitive term 'miscarriage' does not. We have many ways in our culture to avoid the word 'dead', as death is so final. However, as professionals we do have to help parents accept the reality of death and avoid misunderstandings, so it is sometimes appropriate to say 'dead' or 'died'.

If bereavement is what happens to parents then grief is how they feel and react. If bereavement is the wound then grief is the process that follows. It can be painful, take a long time to heal and leave scars. Kubler-Ross's (1970) stages of grief are well known and help illustrate grief as a dynamic process, which the bereaved person must work through.

1. Denial and isolation
2. Confusion or anger
3. Bargaining
4. Depression
5. Acceptance.

However, grief is not a tidy predictable set of reactions. Richard Wilson describes the experience using an analogy of a waterfall (Figure 20.1), suggesting that we row along the river of life unable to see what is ahead. When bereavement occurs he likens the initial shock to the feeling of falling out of control. In this condition parents are unlikely to take in and retain information and certainly may be unable to make important decisions. Grief can be messy and confused and this is illustrated well by the 'whirlpool of grief'. Parents' reactions may be unpredictable, unexpected or sometimes delayed, in this pool they may also clutch at

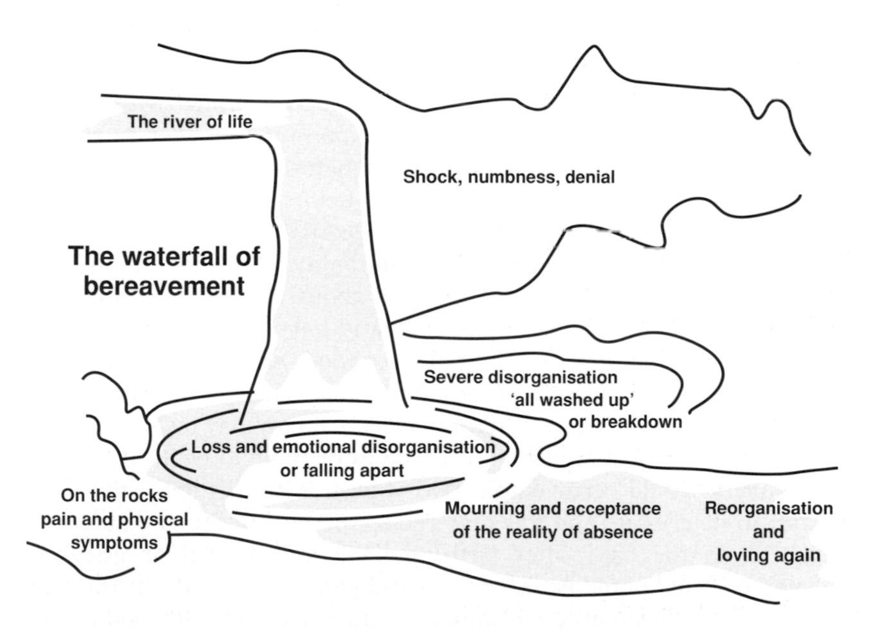

Figure 20.1 The whirlpool of grief (courtesy of Dr Richard Wilson, Consultant Paediatrician, Kingston Hospital, Surrey, UK)

anything that may help keep them afloat. The work of grief uses up energy and can leave the woman feeling lost, lacking confidence and isolated. To help parents grieve professionals need to accept the reality of their suffering and acknowledge the loss of their child (see Making memories).

Breaking the news

There are moments in life that live on, vivid and bright in people's memories. Often a shocking event or being given terrible news is one of those moments. Professionals' words, attitudes and behaviour may stand out in sharp relief against what often becomes a fog of confusion and despair. Thoughtless words, appearing rushed or cold will never be forgotten, but neither will the person who shows kindness, concern and compassion.

When asked, parents often say they knew something was wrong before they were told. It's often better if concerns are shared early with the parents to prepare them. If the baby has died *in utero*, once the diagnosis has been confirmed, parents need to be told honestly and gently, so there can be no doubt. Professional language like 'the fetal heart is absent' or colloquialisms like 'passed away' are inappropriate and a more honest 'I'm sorry but your baby has died ' is probably best.

Intrauterine death

If intrauterine death is suspected this should be confirmed with a real-time ultrasound scan where possible. It is important, however, to ensure that the mother has good support with her when she is told and that after the initial shock she is given plenty of time before being offered options or having to make decisions. It has been suggested that induction within 24 hours may reduce psychological morbidity. However, individual women may have very different feelings about carrying a dead baby. Some women feel they need to go home and have time with their baby to say 'goodbye' preparing for this final separation. A delay of 24–48 hours may give parents this space and they may appreciate the opportunity to see if labour begins naturally. Alternatively, a woman may be distressed at carrying a dead baby and feel it would be intolerable to wait. In 80% of cases delivery would occur within two weeks. With this delay the baby will start to deteriorate and this may reduce parents desire and ability to see and hold the baby after birth, possibly affecting their grieving. However, parents should be listened to and given choices. If it is thought that the baby has been dead for more than three weeks a full blood count, including platelets and clotting studies, should be taken to screen for coagulopathy.

To protect the mothers' health and aid in diagnosing cause of death, one or more of the following tests are often included within local protocols/guidelines:

- Kleihauer
- rhesus antibodies, lupus anticoagulant, anticardiolipin antibody, thrombotic screen
- 'TORCH' screen (or relevant component)
- random blood sugars
- thyroid function.

CARE IN LABOUR

Labour may be when parents start to grieve. Continuity of carers is important and parents need sensitive preparation for what is to come. Some parents need time on their own while others may feel frightened to be left alone. Labour can be a positive experience, the mother may feel this is one thing she can do 'properly'.

PAIN RELIEF

In the past, attempts to take away the pain and 'make things easier' proved to be harmful. Sedation often left the woman confused and detached, delaying and complicating grief. This may still be a risk if heavy doses of opiates are used. Options need to be discussed honestly. Fear, shock and misery may make the pain harder to bear even during early miscarriage. Whatever the stage of pregnancy, good pain relief may help the women feel more in control. Alternatively, giving birth actively with little or no pain relief can empower some women, raise their self-esteem and form part of their memories.

PARTNERS

During labour the woman's partner or supporter is likely to be very anxious about the outcome, with a heightened sense of risk, often demonstrated by increased vigilance. Watching everything that is done, constantly questioning staff and what they are and are not doing is a common reaction to these circumstances. A male partner, who has been socialised into feeling he should be strong and protect his partner, may find being helpless or unable to control the situation frustrating and even unbearable. He may not understand the importance of a vaginal birth to his partner and can become demanding and aggressive. Listening and acknowledging his pain will help. Alternatively, parents often feel protective of others and may make an effort not to upset those around them, including the professional caring for them.

BIRTH

The moment of birth is often very quiet; time seems to be suspended. No matter how long a baby has been dead everyone hopes there has been a terrible mistake. The professional needs to confirm the death: again, a simple 'I'm sorry, the baby is dead' is all that can be said.

During labour, staff should have discussed with parents whether they want to see and hold the baby, what to expect and how the baby may look. Parents may be frightened of seeing a dead body or imagine the abnormal baby as a monster (however, parents generally report that what they imagined was far worse than the reality). In these circumstances they may feel reassured if you hold and look at baby first. Parents appreciate staff who treat the baby with the same care and respect as a live baby. For parents who can hold and touch their baby, the memories they form often help their grieving.

AFTER DELIVERY

At any stage of pregnancy or whatever the circumstances, the intensity of emotions and the speed at which things have happened can be overwhelming. Parents need time with each other and their family to think and talk about what has happened, time to consider decisions and practical arrangements and, if wanted, time with their baby. This may be the only time they have with their child so it should never be rushed. If the parents want to share this time with their family or friends then they should be provided with support and private space in which to do this. If pressures on delivery suite rooms cannot accommodate this, it is better to move parents and their baby to another postnatal room. Many hospitals now provide special 'sanctuary' rooms where the family can be quiet and comfortable. Voluntary organisations are often keen to fund such areas.

Making memories

When a life has been so short it can be very important to create memories.

TIME

For parents whose baby is born dead their first meeting is also a farewell. For many parents being with, seeing and holding their baby will help their grieving. However, parents will have individual needs and they should never feel pressured, only informed and supported. The time parents have with their child is very precious as this is all they will ever have to build their memories and for some this may be the only time they ever have as parents. They should be allowed as much time as they need and never be hurried or rushed (this may be hours and in some cases days). For other parents, the shock and fear of death, religious or cultural reasons may lead them not to hold or even be with their dead baby. All parents should know that this does not have to be their only opportunity and they can always ask to see their baby later.

Over the coming months and years friends and family are going to be the parents main support and if they also have seen and held the baby this will help to confirm the baby's existence and make the grief work easier. Children have often been excluded and protected when there was death in the family. However, if the parents wish and with the right support, involving siblings can be very helpful for the whole family.

PHOTOGRAPHS AND OTHER MEMENTOS

Polaroid photographs have the advantage of being immediate and if a very preterm or ill baby has to be transferred for neonatal care these will help to reduce the parents' sense of separation. Polaroid photographs do fade and discolour and close-up photographs are often of poor quality. Thus, especially when the baby has been born dead, a good 35-mm film should be used. Photographs can be hard to take but are invaluable for many parents working through their grief. Taken with sensitivity and care, these may help parents face the reality of loss even when the baby is very small, damaged or abnormal. In the future parents often become interested in the detail of what their baby looked like. Couples' perceptions of their child's appearance may be very different from that of the professionals. Where we see maceration, discoloration and signs of death, they will see perfect little fingers and toes or grandpa's nose. Parents may appreciate photographs of themselves holding their child or a family picture and when a twin has died often a photograph of the babies together can be comforting (Figure 20.2). Some parents may not wish to see photographs but be willing to have some kept at the hospital for them should they change their minds.

Other mementos, such as handprints or footprints, a lock of hair, cot cards or name bands, can all be created for the parents as keepsakes. Staff should consult and involve parents at this time, for instance, asking whether they would like to cut the baby's hair or where to cut it from, enabling parents to feel more in control and, indeed, more like parents.

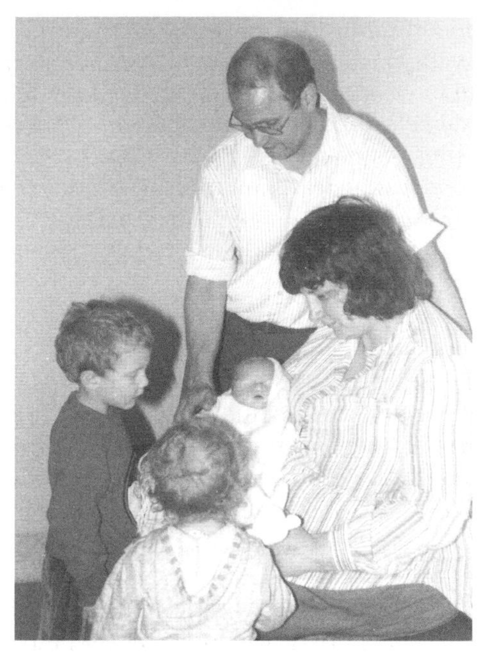

Figure 20.2 The Pearce family with baby Katie who died at one day old (courtesy of the Child Bereavement Trust)

Funeral arrangements

Ensuring that parents have the right information and take time to make decisions about funeral or cremation arrangements is vital. Often this may be the only opportunity for them to share their loss with family and friends and to mark publicly the existence of a baby only they knew. Rushing into a decision to 'let the hospital take care of it all' may be regretted later.

Autopsy

Clearly this needs to be dealt with sensitively providing accurate and clear information. A postmortem examination may help parents to understand what led to their baby's death or whether another pregnancy would carry similar risks. However, they need to know that it may not be able to give them an exact answer to why their baby died. The explanation of the autopsy should be similar to that outlining an operation. The parents should be reassured that if they wish to they can see their baby again (in the case of a baby below 20–22 weeks of gestation, this may not be possible, as the skin is too thin to be resutured). Unfortunately, preparing specimens from young infants sometimes requires that an organ be removed for several weeks. Consent forms should always take into consideration the need for organ removal, retention and disposal.

Thoughtful, accurate completion of the records and a detailed history will aid the pathologist in interpreting the postmortem findings. Parents who do not wish their baby to have an autopsy may be willing for a particular part of the body to be examined or for tissue samples to be taken for chromosome studies. The placenta and membranes should always be sent for investigation.

Cultural sensitivity

Many of us may write down a religion or ethnic background on a form that may reflect little about our individual values, beliefs or preferences. People are unlikely to fit into precise racial stereotypes. Professionals need to be sensitive to parents' cultural backgrounds but never make assumptions about people's beliefs or wishes in relation to death. Individuals may have firm beliefs about how the baby's body should be handled, whether a photograph is appropriate and when, where and how it should be buried or cremated. The only way to get it right is to ask. However, an understanding of peoples' varying philosophies and perspectives can make us more culturally sensitive. The hospital chaplain is likely to be a valuable source of support and information, not just in this area but the whole topic of perinatal loss.

Gender differences

Just as one can never make assumptions about people's religious beliefs and practices, it is impossible to separate out men and women's reactions and try to make generalisations. Each man and woman is an individual and, as indicated at the beginning, the baby will have meant something different to each parent. However, there is much evidence to suggest that men and women are likely to experience different feelings about pregnancy loss or the death of a baby and grieve in a way that is distinctive to them. These can often lead to misunderstandings, feelings of hurt, even betrayal and ultimately conflict between a couple.

Gender roles and stereotyping may be partly to blame for some of these misunderstandings. Men may have grown up in a culture where they were expected to be strong and protective and believe that to show emotion is a sign of weakness. Often professionals reinforce these stereotypical expectations assuming that somehow the father of the baby who has died will be less affected or emotionally distraught than their partner. Staff can support parents in these early days by speaking to them together to strengthen their relationship and reduce misunderstanding and inconsistencies. Encouraging the couple to talk to each other and accept that it is normal to have different feelings will also help.

Special circumstances that may complicate grief

Overall, hospital care of those who experience perinatal loss is evaluated well by parents. However, care is often considered poorer and parents express feelings of confusion due to lack of information in the following circumstances:

- unexplained intrauterine death
- lethal anomaly
- emergency delivery resulting in stillbirth
- the cause of death was preventable.

This would suggest that it is these situations that professionals feel most uncomfortable exploring and less willing to discuss, leaving parents feeling confused and unsupported. Parents who are suddenly and unexpectedly faced with a frightening or traumatic emergency situation will benefit greatly if a member of staff is allocated to stay with them and support them throughout. Listening, debriefing and answering questions will not only aid the grief process and reduce psychological morbidity but can also reduce complaints and litigation.

LATE MISCARRIAGE OR DEATH OF A PRE-24-WEEK FETUS

Late miscarriage of a fetus with no legal status, if not handled sensitively, can lead to increased complications in the parents' grieving. If the baby is not seen or held it may become almost 'invisible' and the lack of formal and informal rituals around registration and funeral arrangements can add to the parents' feelings that their baby did not exist except for them. Whether the baby was pre- or post-24 weeks of gestation makes no difference to how the parents feel, they have still lost their baby. Many hospitals now recognise that this is an issue and are willing to offer a funeral service for babies younger than 24 weeks. Should parents wish to arrange a private burial they will need a letter from a medical practitioner confirming the position.

CONGENITAL ABNORMALITY

Making the decision to terminate a pregnancy for a congenital abnormality can lead to a complex mix of feelings and reactions. Often parents will experience conflicts between their past beliefs and values and the reality of the decision they have to make. Parents have sometimes reported feeling pressured and not being given enough information about their alternatives. Sometimes having made the decision to terminate the pregnancy they feel abandoned by staff, family and friends. Feelings of grief are intense and can become complicated by extreme guilt, sometimes displayed as anger. Guilt may relate to parents feelings of inadequacy at being unable to produce a 'normal' baby and then deciding on termination. Good support and counselling at this time can reduce future problems.

Giving birth to a baby with an unexpected abnormality or disability causes a grief reaction similar to the death of a baby, as the parents mourn the loss of the 'dream baby'. Initial reactions may include shock, numbness and sadness and it is common for parents to express feelings of denial. Parents may reject the baby initially, simply being unable to accept the reality. Occasionally this is a complete rejection and parents decide to have the baby fostered or adopted. Either way, parents will need a huge amount of support. How the news is broken can have long-term effects on the parents' feelings about their baby and its condition. Parents should be informed together and as soon as possible, preferably while they are holding the baby. Use the baby's name if possible and try to use terminology that is sensitive, describes the condition and does not define the baby: for example 'Michael has Down syndrome, not 'He's a Down's baby'. How professionals hold, touch and speak to the baby can have a powerful effect on how parents perceive their baby and the relationships they form.

DEATH OF TWINS AND MULTIPLES

To mourn the death of one baby and celebrate the birth of another baby is a tragic contradiction. Parents may feel unable to celebrate the life of one baby or grieve for the other. This situation means grieving may be delayed and will be complex, possibly leading to long-term psychological and/or relationship problems. Parents should be offered additional support and good quality bereavement counselling.

NEONATAL LOSS

When a baby is seriously ill, parents also demonstrate grief reactions, as they experience the loss of a 'normal' healthy baby. When parents are separated it is vital to keep them informed of the baby's condition and to provide a picture as soon as practical. Parents experience a turmoil of emotions, as each visit to the neonatal unit may bring despair or hope with their baby's changing condition. This leads to high levels of stress and anxiety. Parents may find the technology surrounding their baby frightening and avoid visiting. Some couples, believing that the baby is likely to die, withdraw emotionally in anticipatory mourning. Should the baby survive, this may lead to problems with attachment later. Others may feel ambivalent, wanting the baby to survive against all the odds while at the same time not wanting to see it suffer or survive severely handicapped. It is important to encourage as much contact with the baby as possible to help parents develop a relationship with their baby, which should help them whatever the out come.

Discharge home

Some parents cannot wait to get home and leave the hospital and its painful memories behind. However, many parents may prefer to stay in the hospital for some time, often feeling cocooned and protected from the world outside. This gives them some personal and emotional space before they have to face the outside world. Parents may want to stay close to their baby, either keeping it in the room with them or seeing it regularly. Occasionally, parents may like to take the baby home before the funeral and this should not be discouraged – even though some staff may feel that it is an unusual request.

Before discharge, practical things such as Anti D and rubella status should be checked. As with all postnatal women contraception should be discussed. Talking about sex may seem inappropriate at this time but a couple may seek to comfort each other or reaffirm their feelings for each other through intercourse and an unplanned pregnancy would be likely to complicate grief considerably. Literature on perinatal loss is valuable, as it may reinforce many of the things they have been told but were unable to take in earlier. Contact details for support groups such as SANDS (the Stillbirth and Neonatal Death Society) should be included in the literature, as they may be appreciated later.

Parents should always be given an appointment to come back to discuss the autopsy and other investigations as soon as possible and this may be earlier than the traditional six weeks. In the meantime, in case they have any questions, contact numbers for senior staff should be provided. At the follow-up consultation endeavour to see both parents together, ensure that you refer to the baby using the correct sex and by name whenever possible. Again, listening is vital and often information has to be repeated that parents may have not been able to absorb after the baby's death. Good communication on discharge is vital to avoid unnecessary pain: details such as cancellation of antenatal appointments and informing the community midwife, family doctor and health visitor of the babies death are essential.

Pregnancy following a loss

If possible, couples should be encouraged to wait 12 months before a further pregnancy to reduce the risks of depression. For a third-trimester loss the World Health Organization recommends at least 18 months. This wait provides time for both emotional and physical regeneration and optimises the woman's preconceptual health and nutritional status. Clearly the next pregnancy is going to be a difficult time. Mothers are going to feel anxious, scared and nervous, which will be mentally, emotionally and physically taxing. To protect themselves from more pain they are likely to try to remain detached from their developing baby. Parental anxiety can be greatly relieved by early consultation. What parents appreciate most is someone who is willing to listen to their story and understand how they feel.

Improving the quality of care

Perinatal loss involves doctors, midwives, nurses, chaplains and support staff working together to provide the best quality care for parents. In order to do this effectively, staff should have appropriate education and training in dealing with perinatal loss. They also need to work in an environment where they feel supported and each unit should have a system that enables staff to debrief after being involved in perinatal loss.

Good management of perinatal loss involves many team members and can often appear complex. It helps to have good comprehensive guidelines and even a checklist that is reviewed regularly. However, this should only be used as a guide and never as a systematic strategy or list of tasks that does not allow for sensitively meeting the individual needs of parents. Professionals need to communicate well, develop protocols and regularly audit the service they offer.

Best practice on perinatal loss is not complex or technical and often the changes needed to ensure good service are simple and need few resources. It is important to get the care right because to get it wrong can do a great deal of harm to parents and families.

Reference

Kubler-Ross E. (1970) *On Death and Dying*. New York: Macmillan.

Further reading

Chambers HM, Chan FY. (1999) Support for women and families after perinatal death. *Cochrane Database Syst Rev* (2)

Enkins M, Keirse M, Neilson J, Crowther C, Duley L, Hodnett E, Hofmeyer J. Fetal death. In: *A Guide to Effective Care in Pregnancy and Childbirth,* 3rd ed. Oxford: Oxford University Press. p. 240–4.

Fox R, Pillai M. (2000) The management of intrauterine death. In: Kean L, Baker P, Edelstone D. *Best Practice in Labour Ward Management.* Edinburgh: WB Saunders. p. 337–62.

Gilbert ES, Harman JS. (1998) Pregnancy loss and perinatal grief. In: *Manual of High Risk Pregnancy and Delivery.* 2nd ed. London: Mosby. p. 133–83.

Mander R. (1994) *Loss and Bereavement in Childbearing.* London: Blackwell Scientific.

Royal College of Obstetricians and Gynaecologists, Royal College of Pathologists. (2001) *Fetal and Perinatal Pathology: Report of a Joint Working Party.* London: RCOG Press.

SANDS. (1995) *Guidelines for Professionals on Pregnancy Loss and the Death of a Baby.* 2nd ed. London: Stillbirth and Neonatal Death Society.

Index

Paediatric and Adolescent Gynaecology for the MRCOG and Beyond

Anne Garden and Joanne Topping

A broad knowledge of caring for children and adolescents with gynaecological disorders is essential for everyone in clinical practice. All clinicians, at some point in their careers, will be required to deal with young people who present with symptoms that could possibly be due to gynaecological pathology. This book covers the whole range of developments in the field of paediatric and adolescent gynaecology, ranging from conditions specific to childhood to contraception, female genital mutilation and gynaecological malignancies. The subject is dealt with in a sensitive and understanding manner and is clearly written by authors with a worldwide reputation in the field. It is an invaluable aid, not only for candidates preparing to sit the MRCOG examination but also for those in clinical practice, midwives and, indeed, any health professional who comes into contact with young people.

Contents: Preface; Pubertal growth and development; Indeterminate genitalia; Gynaecological problems in childhood; Endocrine disorders; Child sexual abuse; Amenorrhoea; Menstrual problems in teenagers; Contraception; Female genital mutilation; Gynaecological tumours; Index.

1-900364-42-5 | 96 pages | Published 2001

Antenatal Disorders for the MRCOG and Beyond

Andrew Thompson and Ian Greer

Patterns and provision of antenatal care have changed enormously in recent years in response to the opinions of consumers, providers, professional associations and government reports. During pregnancy, most women remain well and require little formal medical input. For them, pregnancy is a physiological process. However, some women develop complications with significant morbidity or mortality for their baby and, occasionally, for themselves. Providers of antenatal care must be able to distinguish between these two groups of women and arrange with them an appropriate and personalised plan of care.

Contents: Preface; Antenatal care and risk assessment; Assessment of fetal growth and well-being; Antepartum haemorrhage; Multiple pregnancy; Preterm labour; Hypertensive disorders of pregnancy; Common medical disorders in pregnancy; Rhesus disease; Recommended reading; Index.

1-900364-36-0 | 208 pages | Published 2000

Management of Infertility for the MRCOG and Beyond

Allan Templeton, P Ashok, S Bhattacharya, R Gazvani, M Hamilton, S MacMillan & A Shetty

Every MRCOG candidate must have a broad knowledge of infertility management. This volume has been written jointly by members of one of the most prestigious infertility clinics in the UK (Aberdeen Maternity Hospital) and provides information on all aspects of infertility, both male and female.

Contents: Preface; The management of infertility; The initial assessment of the infertile couple; Male factor infertility; Disorders of ovulation; Tubal-factor infertility; Infertility and endometriosis; Unexplained infertility; Assisted conception techniques; Glossary; Recommended reading; Index.

1-900364-29-8 | 131 pages | Published 2000

Gynaecological and Obstetric Pathology for the MRCOG

Harold Fox and Hilary Buckley

This succinct and copiously illustrated volume covers pathological conditions of the vulva, vagina, uterus, fallopian tube and ovary, in addition to abnormalities related to pregnancy, and cervical cytology. Gynaecological and Obstetric Pathology is an invaluable revision text for candidates preparing for the Part 1 and Part 2 MRCOG Examination, and is in addition a readily accessible, concise and up-to-date reference text for practising clinicians.

Contents: Preface; The vulva; The vagina; The cervix; The endometrium; The myometrium; The fallopian tube; The ovary; Abnormalities related to pregnancy; Cervical cytology, *by Dulcie V Coleman*; Suggested references for further reading; Index.

0-902331-84-1 184 pages 1998

Menstrual Problems for the MRCOG

Mary Anne Lumsden, Jane Norman and Hilary Critchley

This text covers normal endometrial function, evaluation of the uterine cavity, medical and surgical treatment of menstrual problems, dysmenorrhoea, adolescent bleeding problems, perimenopausal and iatrogenic bleeding.

Contents: Preface; Introduction; Normal endometrial function; Evaluation of the uterine cavity; Medical management of menstrual problems; Surgical treatment of menstrual problems; Dysmenorrhoea; Adolescent bleeding problems; Iatrogenic bleeding; Index.

0-902331-83-3 111 pages Published 1997

Neonatology for the MRCOG

Peter Dear and Simon Newell

Written with the trainee obstetrician in mind and concentrates on those aspects of the subject that are relevant to obstetric decision making.

Contents: Preface; Introduction; The effects of birth on the fetus; Care of the normal infant; The preterm infant; Intrauterine growth retardation; Nutrition and infant feeding; Jaundice; Common congenital abnormalities; Infection of the fetus and newborn; Blood disorders; Hydrops fetalis; Inborn errors of metabolism; Neonatal effects of maternal disease; Suggested references for further reading; Index.

0-902331-82-5 136 pages Published 1996

The MRCOG: A Guide to the Examination

IR Johnson, IT Cameron, EJ Owen, P Bowen-Simpkins and JM Rymer

An essential up-to-date guide to the Examination and gives full details of recent changes in its structure and regulations. Examples of questions and model answers, helpful hints, together with the complete syllabus and suggested reading list mean that this book should be at the top of any candidate's shopping list. Covers both Part 1 and Part 2 examinations.

1-900364-28-X 60 pages Published 2000